HASHIMOTO'S DIET COOKBOOK FOR BEGINNERS

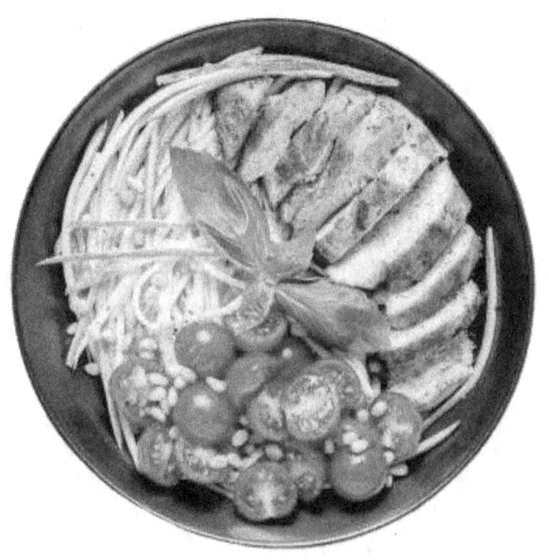

Easy Nutritious Healing Recipes to Reset Hyperthyroidism and Boost Overall Well-Being

Joan G. Milone

Copyright © 2024 by Joan G. Milone
All rights reserved.

No part of this book may be reproduced, stored in a retrieval system, or transmitted in any form or by any means, electronic, mechanical, photocopying, recording, or otherwise, without prior written permission of the copyright owner.

This book is written as a source of information only. The information contained in this book is provided in good faith and is believed to be accurate and reliable as of the date of publication. The author does not assume any responsibility for any errors or omissions that may appear.

Table of Contents

Table of Contents

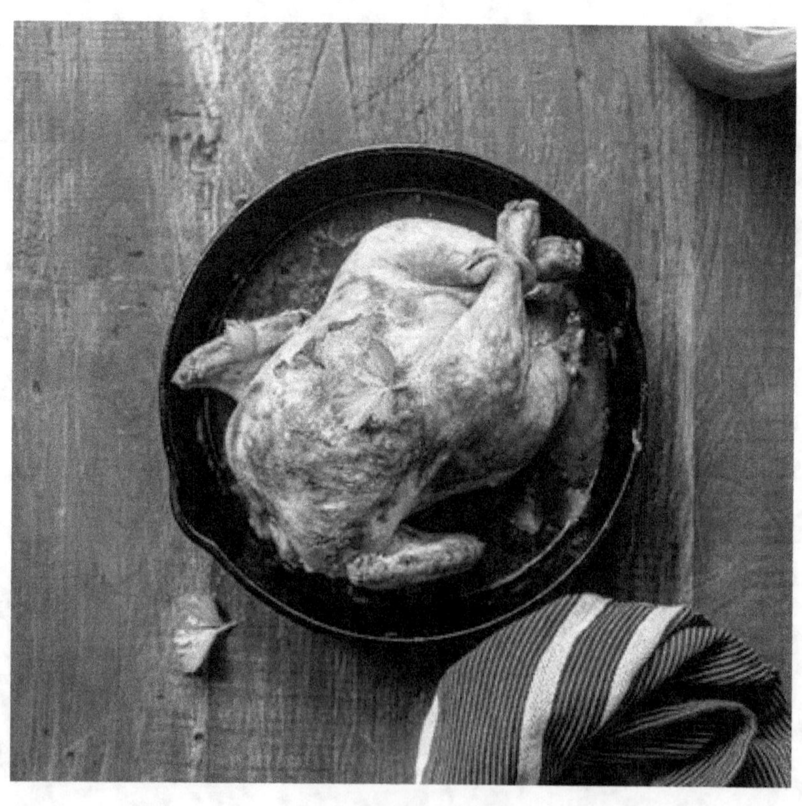

INTRODUCTION

In the early hours of the morning, as the world awakens, there is a promise—a promise of new beginnings, days full of vigor, and a life reclaimed from the shadows of Hashimoto's illness. This is more than simply a recipe; it's a light of hope for those who have walked through the fog of doubt and long for a road to health. Welcome to the "Hashimoto's Diet Cookbook for Beginners," where each recipe represents a new chapter in your journey to health and restoration.

Our story begins in the present, with you, rather than once upon a time. Hashimoto's, a silent opponent disguised as an autoimmune condition, has tested many, transforming their bodies into battlegrounds. But what if I told you that there is a weapon during this war that is both powerful and nurturing, with the potential to turn the tide? This weapon does not shine with steel; rather, it gleams with the hues of nature, the perfume of spices, and the warmth of a home-cooked dinner.

This is your invitation to go on a culinary journey unlike any other— one in which the kitchen serves as your laboratory and food becomes more than just nutrition; it becomes a health ally. "Understanding Hashimoto's Disease" is our beginning point, revealing the secrets of your foe and building the groundwork for the adventure ahead.

As you read these pages, you'll learn more than simply recipes; you'll also discover secrets to breaking the chains of symptoms that have kept you back. Each dish has been meticulously designed not just to please your palate, but also to nourish your body and soul, gently guiding you toward a state of equilibrium and health.

So, join me. Let's stir, chop, and cook our way to well-being. Let's see each meal as a time to heal, celebrate, and love. Your journey to a better, happier self begins now, and it will be delightful.

Understanding Hashimoto's Disease

Hashimoto's disease, an autoimmune illness, develops when the immune system erroneously attacks the thyroid gland, resulting in chronic thyroid underactivity or hypothyroidism. This tiny gland in the neck produces hormones that control metabolism, energy, and mood. When Hashimoto's disease impairs its function, it can cause a variety of symptoms, including weight gain, weariness, mood fluctuations, and sensitivity to cold.

Understanding Hashimoto's is critical since it involves not only controlling symptoms but also addressing the underlying cause: an immune system in disarray. The disease frequently progresses slowly, and its symptoms might be confused with those of other conditions, making early discovery and care critical. In addition to medical treatment, diet, and lifestyle changes play an important part in Hashimoto's disease management. Certain foods can help reduce inflammation and improve thyroid function, whilst others might aggravate symptoms.

Understanding Hashimoto's requires recognizing it as more than a thyroid problem; it is an immune system challenge that impacts the entire body. Knowledge enables people to take proactive actions towards wellness, changing their attitudes around diet, stress management, and self-care, laying the groundwork for a healthy life despite the disease.

How to Use This Cookbook

1. **Familiarize Yourself with Hashimoto's**: Begin by reading the introductory sections that explain Hashimoto's disease and its impact on your health. Understanding the connection between your diet and thyroid function is crucial for making the most out of this cookbook.

2. **Plan Your Meals**: Use the recipes and meal planning templates provided to start planning your meals. Consider your personal preferences, dietary restrictions, and the nutritional insights shared in the book to create balanced meals that support thyroid health.

3. **Shop Smart**: Equip yourself with the shopping lists tailored for Hashimoto's-friendly ingredients. Focus on whole, unprocessed foods, and be mindful of any personal food sensitivities. These lists are designed to make grocery shopping easier and healthier.

4. **Cook with Intention**: As you explore the recipes, cook with the intention of nourishing your body. Each recipe is crafted not just for flavor, but to provide the nutrients essential for managing Hashimoto's. Pay attention to the tips on how to adjust recipes to suit your taste and nutritional needs.

5. **Reflect and Adjust**: Lastly, pay attention to how your body responds to the changes in your diet. Reflect on your progress and how different foods affect your symptoms. Feel free to adjust and experiment with the recipes to better suit your body's needs. This cookbook is not just a guide but a tool for personal discovery and healing.

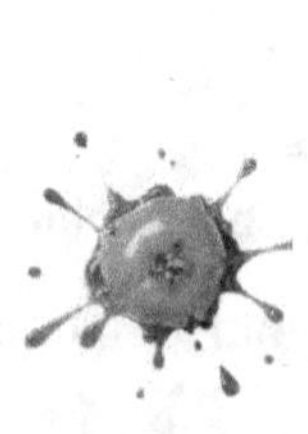
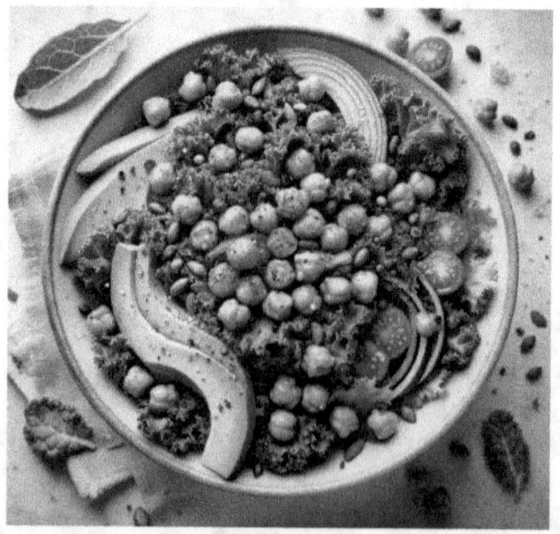
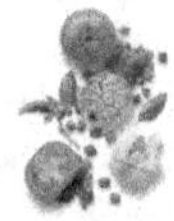

CHAPTER 1: THE BASICS OF THE HASHIMOTO'S DIET

Exploring "The Basics of the Hashimoto's Diet" is the first step toward a more balanced and healthier lifestyle. This part is about knowing how to eat in a way that benefits your thyroid and calms your immune system. You'll discover the benefits of healthy, anti-inflammatory foods and learn how to customize your diet to your body's specific requirements. It's all about empowerment—giving you the knowledge and recipes you need to make healthier choices. Let's go on this trip together, converting your eating habits into a route to health and vitality.

Key Nutrients for Hashimoto's

Navigating Hashimoto's disease necessitates a deliberate approach to nutrition, with a focus on important nutrients that promote thyroid health and immunological function. Here's a brief look at vital nutrients that can help persons with Hashimoto's:

Selenium: This trace mineral is essential in the conversion of thyroid hormones from inactive to active forms. Foods high in selenium, such as Brazil nuts, sunflower seeds, and shellfish, are excellent choices for your diet.

Zinc: Zinc is essential for thyroid hormone synthesis and helps to maintain appropriate thyroid function. Beef, chicken, and beans are excellent sources.

Iron: Iron deficiency can worsen thyroid function. Iron-rich foods such as spinach, lentils, and red meat can help you maintain appropriate levels.

Omega-3 Fatty Acids: These fats are essential for reducing inflammation and supporting immune system balance. Fatty fish, flaxseeds, and walnuts are great sources.

Vitamin D: Vitamin D is often inadequate in Hashimoto's patients; however, it is essential for immunological control. Aside from sunlight exposure, consider fatty fish and fortified foodstuffs.

B Vitamins: Particularly B12 and B6 are important for energy and overall metabolic health. They can be found in meat, fish, eggs, and dairy products.

Incorporating these foods into your diet can help control Hashimoto's symptoms and promote thyroid function. Remember, the goal is to create a well-balanced diet that nourishes your body while also meeting your specific demands.

Foods to Eat and Avoid

When managing Hashimoto's, understanding which foods to embrace and which to minimize can make a significant difference in how you feel. Here's a straightforward guide:

Foods to Eat:

1. **Anti-inflammatory Foods**: Focus on fruits, vegetables, and omega-3 rich foods like salmon, chia seeds, and flaxseeds to combat inflammation.

2. **Selenium-Rich Foods**: Brazil nuts, sunflower seeds, and mushrooms can support thyroid function.

3. **High-Iron Foods**: Include spinach, lentils, and fortified cereals to avoid iron deficiency.

4. **Whole Grains**: Opt for gluten-free grains like quinoa, rice, and oats to maintain energy levels.

5. **Lean Proteins**: Chicken, turkey, and legumes provide necessary nutrients without overwhelming the thyroid.

6. **Healthy Fats**: Avocado, olive oil, and nuts offer healthy fats for overall wellness.

Foods to Avoid:

1. **Gluten**: Many with Hashimoto's find gluten can aggravate symptoms; opting for gluten-free options may help.

2. **Soy**: Soy products can interfere with thyroid hormone absorption and are best minimized.

3. **Excessive Iodine**: While necessary in small amounts, too much iodine can exacerbate thyroid issues.

4. **Processed Foods**: High in unhealthy fats, sugars, and chemicals, these can increase inflammation.

5. **Goitrogens in Excess**: Foods like cabbage, broccoli, and kale, when eaten in large quantities, especially raw, can affect thyroid function. Cooking these foods can reduce their goitrogenic effect.

6. **Sugary Foods and Drinks**: These can spike energy levels temporarily but lead to fatigue and mood swings.

By focusing on nutrient-rich, whole foods and minimizing inflammatory and processed foods, you can support your thyroid health and potentially reduce Hashimoto's symptoms.

Managing Your Diet: A Daily Guide

Managing your diet with Hashimoto's involves mindful eating and planning to support thyroid health and overall wellness. Here's a daily guide to help you navigate your meals and snacks:

Morning Ritual:

- Start with a glass of water to hydrate your body after a night's rest. Consider adding lemon for a vitamin C boost.

- Breakfast: Opt for a balanced meal with protein, healthy fats, and fiber. A smoothie with spinach, berries, a scoop of protein powder, and flaxseed oil can kickstart your day.

Mid-Morning Snack:

- Choose a snack that's rich in protein and healthy fats to maintain energy levels. A small handful of Brazil nuts or an apple with almond butter are great options.

Lunch:

- Focus on a hearty, balanced meal. A salad with mixed greens, grilled chicken, avocado, and a variety of vegetables, dressed with olive oil and lemon juice, supports both digestion and energy levels through the afternoon.

Afternoon Snack:

- To avoid the afternoon energy slump, snack on something light yet satisfying. Carrot sticks with hummus or a piece of fruit are perfect for a quick pick-me-up.

Dinner:

- Keep dinner balanced and lighter than lunch. Fish like salmon, rich in omega-3 fatty acids, served with steamed broccoli and quinoa, offers a nutrient-dense end to the day.

Evening Ritual:

- A small, nutritious snack an hour before bed can help maintain blood sugar levels through the night. A warm cup of herbal tea with a slice of turkey or a small, ripe banana can be soothing.

General Tips:

- Hydration is key. Aim for 8-10 glasses of water throughout the day to support digestion and overall health.

- Listen to your body. If you're feeling full, save the rest for later. If you're still hungry, add more non-starchy vegetables or lean protein to your meals.

- Meal prep can save time and stress. Preparing meals and snacks in advance ensures you have healthy options readily available.

This daily guide is not one-size-fits-all; adjust it based on your activity level, dietary needs, and how different foods make you feel. With time and attention, you can create a diet plan that supports your health and fits your lifestyle.

CHAPTER 2: BREAKFAST AND SMOOTHIES

Breakfast is frequently referred to as the most important meal of the day, and for people dealing with Hashimoto's, this couldn't be more true. It sets the tone for your energy, emotions, and metabolic rate. In this section, we'll look at how to create the ideal morning meals that not only satisfy your taste buds but also benefit your thyroid and general health. Smoothies, in example, are a versatile and tasty way to pack a range of nutrients into a single glass, ensuring that you start your day on the right track.

Sunrise Smoothie

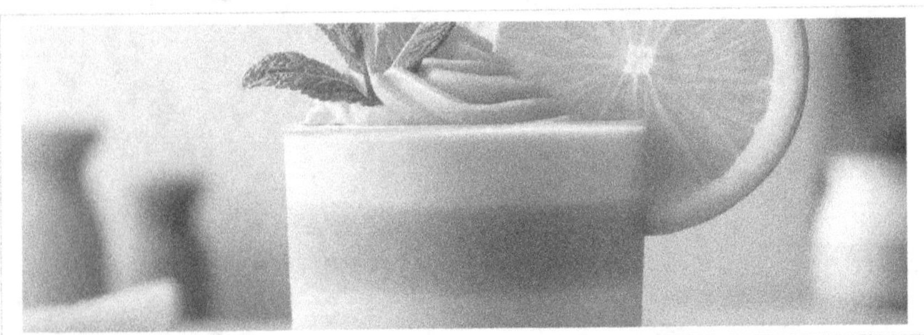

Ingredients:

- 1 cup fresh orange juice
- 1/2 cup frozen raspberries
- 1/2 cup frozen mango chunks
- 1 banana
- 1/2 teaspoon grated ginger
- Ice cubes (optional)

Preparation:

1. In a blender, combine the orange juice, raspberries, mango, banana, and ginger.
2. Blend on high until smooth. If the smoothie is too thick, you can add a little water or more orange juice to reach your desired consistency.
3. Taste and adjust the sweetness, adding a bit of honey if needed.
4. Serve immediately, garnished with a slice of orange and a sprig of mint for that extra touch.

Nutritional Values:

- Calories: 220 kcal
- Protein: 3 g
- Carbohydrates: 55 g
- Fat: 1 g
- Fiber: 7 g
- Vitamin C: 130% of the RDI

Cooking Time: 5 minutes

Serves: 2

Rating: ★★★★★

This Sunrise Smoothie is the perfect way to start your day with a burst of energy and a touch of tropical bliss.

Avocado Toast with Poached Egg

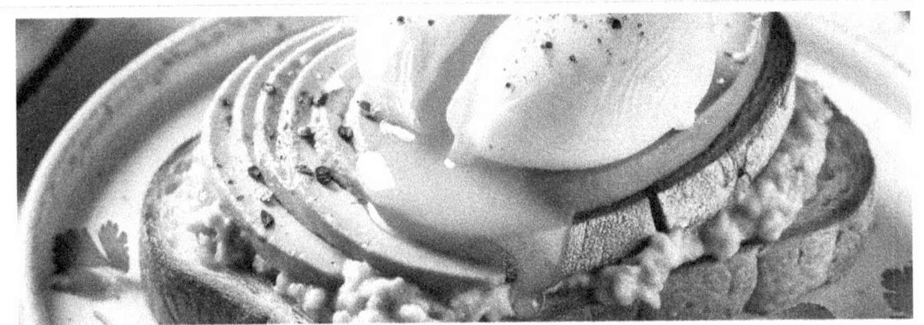

Ingredients:

- 1 large egg
- 1 slice whole grain bread
- 1/2 ripe avocado
- Salt and pepper to taste
- Chili flakes (optional)
- Fresh cilantro (optional)

Preparation:

1. Toast the slice of whole grain bread to your liking.
2. Smash the avocado in a bowl and season with salt and pepper. Spread evenly over the toast.
3. Poach the egg: Bring a pot of water to a light simmer, add a splash of vinegar, create a whirlpool, and gently drop the egg in. Cook for 3-4 minutes, then remove with a slotted spoon.
4. Place the poached egg on top of the avocado toast. Season with chili flakes, fresh cracked black pepper, and garnish with cilantro.

Nutritional Values:

- Calories: 300 kcal
- Protein: 12 g
- Carbohydrates: 30 g

Cooking Time: 10 minutes

Serves: 1   **Rating:** ★★★★★

- Fat: 16 g
- Fiber: 7 g

This Avocado Toast with Poached Egg combines creamy avocado and a runny egg on crunchy toast, making it a wholesome, satisfying start to your day.

Quinoa Porridge with Berries

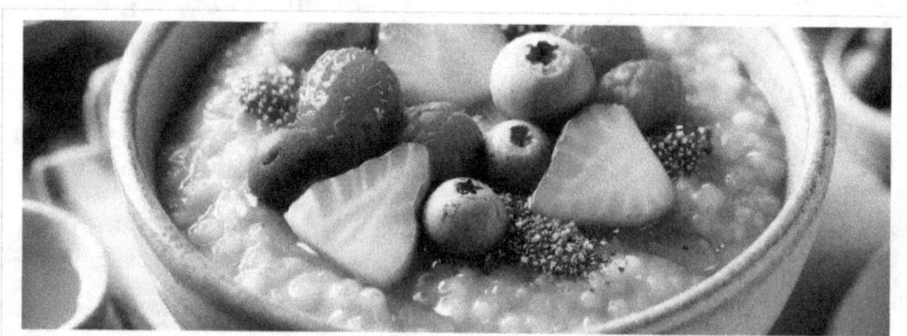

Ingredients:

- 1 cup cooked quinoa
- 1 cup almond milk (or any milk of choice)
- 1/2 teaspoon vanilla extract
- 1 tablespoon honey (or to taste)
- 1/2 cup mixed berries (strawberries, blueberries, raspberries)
- A pinch of cinnamon (optional)

Preparation:

1. In a small pot, combine the cooked quinoa and almond milk. Heat over medium heat until warm.

2. Stir in the vanilla extract and a pinch of cinnamon, if using.

3. Once the mixture is heated through and begins to thicken slightly, remove from heat.

4. Pour the porridge into a bowl, top with mixed berries, and drizzle with honey.

Nutritional Values:

- Calories: 285 kcal
- Protein: 8 g
- Carbohydrates: 50 g
- Fat: 5 g
- Fiber: 5 g

Cooking Time: 10 minutes

Serves: 1   **Rating:** ★★★★★

This Quinoa Porridge with Berries offers a delightful and nutritious start to your day, combining the health benefits of quinoa with the sweetness and antioxidants of fresh berries.

Spinach and Mushroom Omelette

Ingredients:

- 2 large eggs
- 1/4 cup sliced mushrooms
- 1/4 cup fresh spinach
- Salt and pepper to taste

- 1 tablespoon olive oil
- Sliced cherry tomatoes for garnish

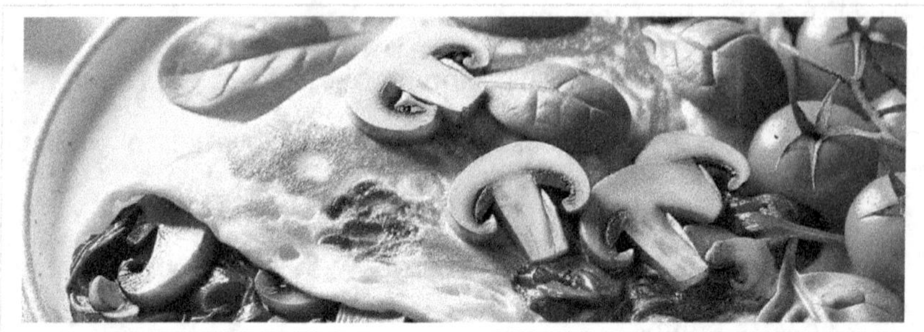

Preparation:

1. Heat olive oil in a pan over medium heat. Add mushrooms and sauté until they begin to brown.
2. Add spinach to the pan and cook until wilted. Remove from pan and set aside.
3. In a bowl, beat the eggs with salt and pepper.
4. Pour the eggs into the pan, tilting to spread evenly. Cook until the edges start to lift from the pan.
5. Place the mushroom and spinach mixture over half of the omelette. Carefully fold the other half over the filling.
6. Serve on a plate, garnished with sliced cherry tomatoes and a few fresh spinach leaves.

Nutritional Values:

- Calories: 250 kcal
- Protein: 14 g
- Carbohydrates: 4 g
- Fat: 20 g

- Fiber: 1 g

Cooking Time: 15 minutes

Serves: 1   **Rating:** ★★★★★

This Spinach and Mushroom Omelette is a delicious and nutritious way to start your day, packed with protein and veggies for a fulfilling breakfast.

Chia Seed Pudding

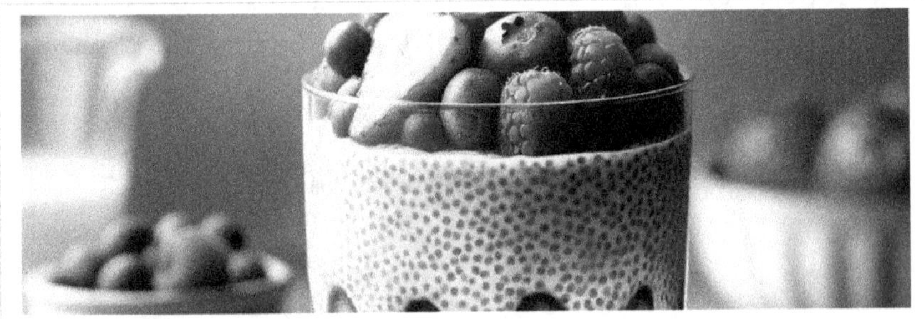

Ingredients:

- 1/4 cup chia seeds
- 1 cup almond milk (or any milk of your choice)
- 1 tablespoon maple syrup (or to taste)
- 1/2 teaspoon vanilla extract
- Fresh mixed berries (strawberries, blueberries, raspberries) for topping

Preparation:

1. In a mixing bowl, combine chia seeds, almond milk, maple syrup, and vanilla extract. Stir well.
2. Cover the bowl and refrigerate for at least 4 hours, or overnight, until the mixture achieves a pudding-like consistency.
3. Once set, give the pudding a good stir to break up any clumps.
4. Serve in a clear glass, topped with a generous layer of fresh mixed berries.

Nutritional Values:

- Calories: 200 kcal
- Protein: 5 g
- Carbohydrates: 24 g
- Fat: 10 g
- Fiber: 10 g

Cooking Time: 5 minutes preparation + chilling time

Serves: 1

Rating: ★★★★★

Chia Seed Pudding is a simple yet elegant breakfast or snack, offering a nutritious blend of omega-3 fatty acids, fiber, and protein, beautifully complemented by the natural sweetness of fresh berries.

Banana Almond Smoothie

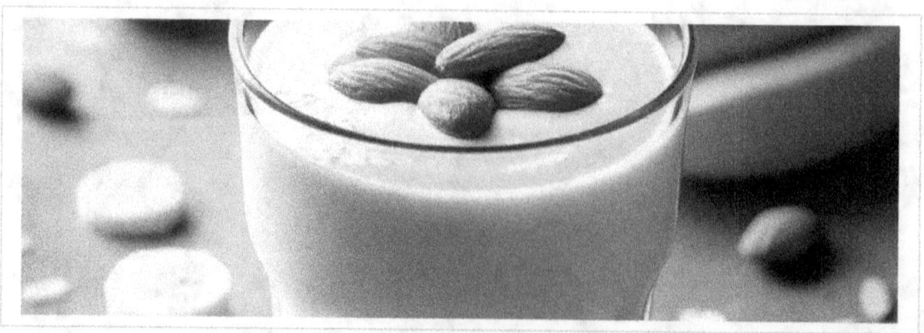

Ingredients:

- 1 ripe banana
- 1 cup almond milk
- 2 tablespoons almond butter
- 1 tablespoon honey (optional)
- A handful of ice cubes
- Sliced almonds for garnish

Preparation:

1. Combine the banana, almond milk, almond butter, honey (if using), and ice cubes in a blender.
2. Blend until smooth and creamy.
3. Pour into a tall glass and garnish with sliced almonds.

Nutritional Values:

- Calories: 320 kcal
- Protein: 8 g
- Carbohydrates: 44 g
- Fat: 14 g
- Fiber: 6 g

Cooking Time: 5 minutes

Serves: 1

Rating: ★★★★★

This Banana Almond Smoothie is the perfect blend of nutty and sweet, offering a delicious and nourishing way to start your day or refuel after a workout.

Sweet Potato Hash

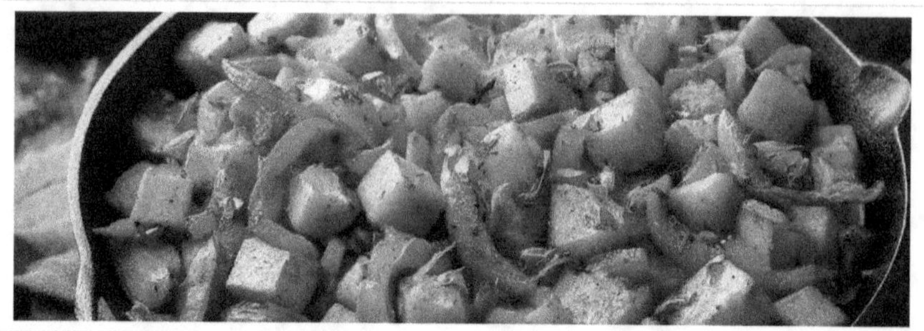

Ingredients:

- 2 large sweet potatoes, peeled and diced
- 1 red bell pepper, diced
- 1 medium onion, diced
- 2 tablespoons olive oil
- Salt and pepper to taste
- Fresh herbs (such as parsley or thyme) for garnish

Preparation:

1. Heat olive oil in a large skillet over medium heat.
2. Add the diced sweet potatoes to the skillet, stirring occasionally, until they start to soften, about 10 minutes.
3. Mix in the diced red bell pepper and onion. Continue to cook, stirring occasionally, until the vegetables are tender and the edges of the sweet potatoes are crispy, about 10 more minutes.
4. Season with salt and pepper to taste. Garnish with fresh herbs before serving.

Nutritional Values:

- Calories: 220 kcal per serving
- Protein: 3 g
- Carbohydrates: 40 g
- Fat: 7 g
- Fiber: 6 g

Cooking Time: 20 minutes

Serves: 4

Rating: ★★★★★

This Sweet Potato Hash is a colorful and nutritious dish, perfect for a comforting breakfast or brunch. Its blend of sweet and savory flavors, combined with a satisfying crunch, makes it a beloved favorite.

Berry Bliss Smoothie

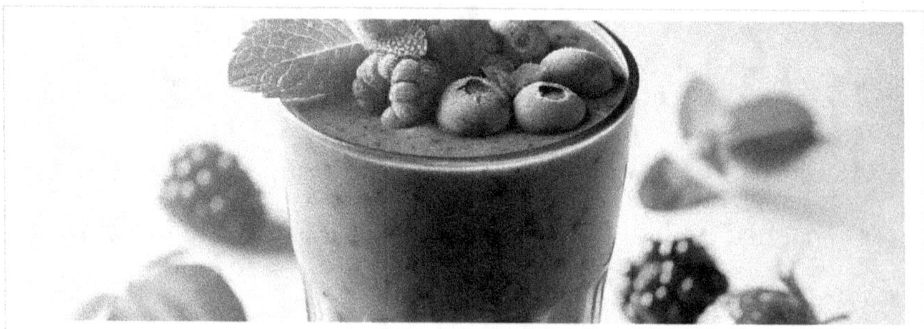

Ingredients:

- 1/2 cup strawberries
- 1/2 cup blueberries
- 1/2 cup raspberries
- 1/2 cup blackberries
- 1 cup almond milk (or milk of choice)
- 1 tablespoon honey (optional)
- Ice cubes (optional)

Preparation:

1. Combine all berries, almond milk, and honey (if using) in a blender. Add ice cubes for a colder smoothie, if desired.
2. Blend until smooth and creamy.
3. Pour into a tall glass and garnish with a mint leaf and a few whole berries on the side.

Nutritional Values:

- Calories: 180 kcal
- Protein: 3 g
- Carbohydrates: 38 g
- Fat: 2 g
- Fiber: 10 g

Cooking Time: 5 minutes

Serves: 2

Rating: ★★★★★

This Berry Bliss Smoothie is a delightful blend of sweet and tart flavors, packed with antioxidants and vitamins. It's the perfect way to start your day or enjoy as a refreshing snack.

Coconut Yogurt Parfait

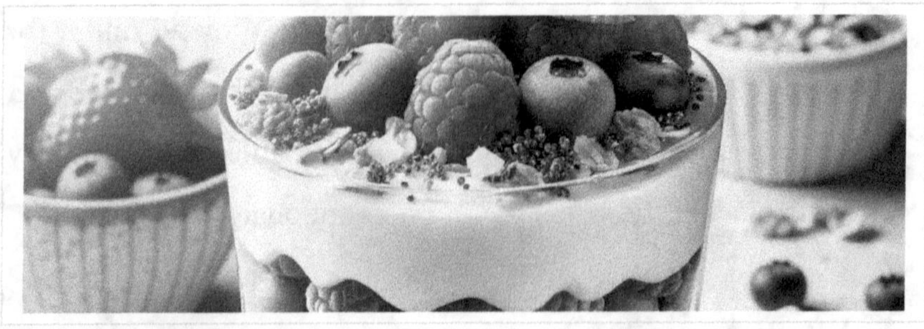

Ingredients:

- 1 cup coconut yogurt
- 1/2 cup mixed berries (strawberries, blueberries, raspberries)
- 1/2 cup granola
- Optional garnishes: mint leaf, chia seeds

Preparation:

1. In a clear glass, layer half of the coconut yogurt at the bottom.
2. Add a layer of mixed berries over the yogurt.
3. Add a layer of granola for crunch.
4. Repeat the layers if desired or if your glass allows, finishing with a layer of berries or granola.
5. Garnish with a mint leaf and a sprinkle of chia seeds for extra flavor and nutrition.

Nutritional Values:

- Calories: 350 kcal
- Protein: 8 g
- Carbohydrates: 45 g
- Fat: 16 g (varies with the type of granola used)
- Fiber: 6 g

Cooking Time: 5 minutes

Serves: 1

Rating: ★★★★★

This Coconut Yogurt Parfait offers a delightful combination of creamy yogurt, fresh berries, and crunchy granola, making it a perfect breakfast or snack that's not only delicious but also nourishing.

Apple Cinnamon Oatmeal

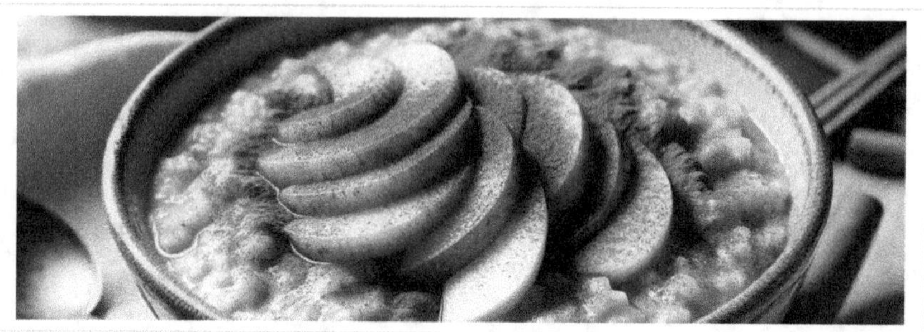

Ingredients:

- 1 cup rolled oats
- 2 cups water or milk
- 1 apple, peeled and diced
- 1/2 teaspoon ground cinnamon
- 1 tablespoon honey or maple syrup
- A pinch of salt

Preparation:

1. In a saucepan, bring water or milk to a boil. Add the oats and a pinch of salt, then reduce the heat to simmer.

2. Cook the oats, stirring occasionally, until they have absorbed the liquid and are fully cooked, about 5 minutes.

3. While the oats are cooking, sauté the diced apple in a separate pan with cinnamon until soft and fragrant.

4. Stir the cooked apples and honey (or maple syrup) into the oatmeal.

5. Serve warm, topped with additional cinnamon or apple slices if desired.

Nutritional Values:

- Calories: 300 kcal
- Protein: 10 g
- Carbohydrates: 55 g
- Fat: 5 g
- Fiber: 8 g

Cooking Time: 10 minutes

Serves: 2   **Rating:** ★★★★★

This Apple Cinnamon Oatmeal is the epitome of a cozy and comforting breakfast, combining the heartiness of oats with the sweet warmth of cinnamon apples. It's a nutritious and delicious way to start your day.

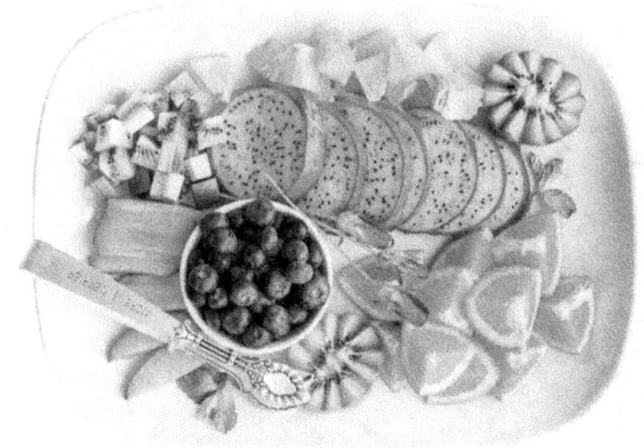

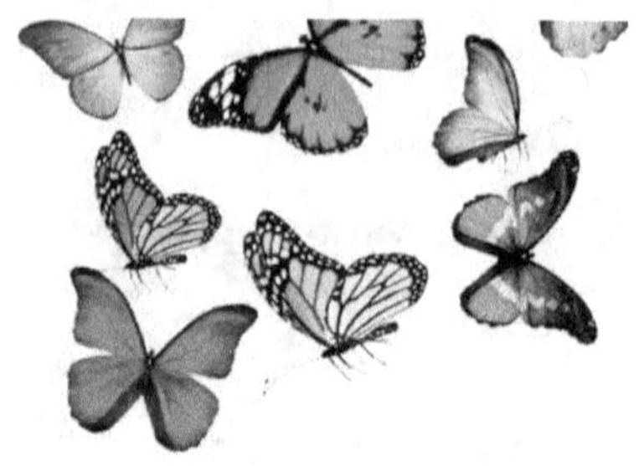

"Every healthy meal is a step toward a happier thyroid. Keep going, your body thanks you for each nutritious choice that supports balance and well-being."

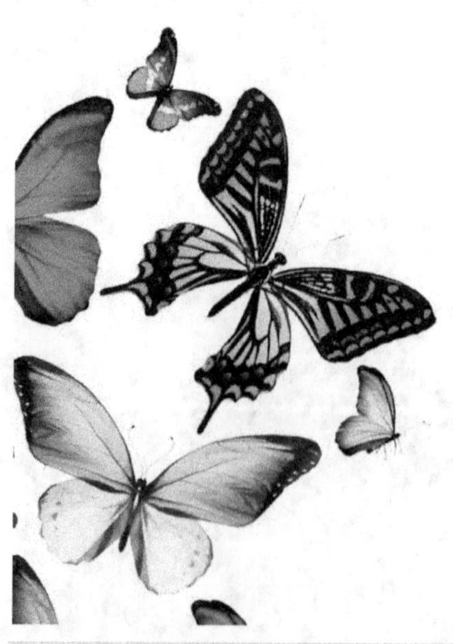

CHAPTER 3: LUNCH

Lunch, the midday pause that recharges our bodies and minds, is more than just a meal—it's an opportunity to nourish ourselves with foods that sustain our energy through the afternoon. In this section, we explore lunches that are not only delightful to the palate but also kind to your body, especially for those managing Hashimoto's. From vibrant salads and hearty soups to satisfying wraps and bowls, each recipe is crafted with ingredients that support thyroid health and overall well-being. Whether you're at home, at work, or on the go, these lunch ideas are designed to be both practical and delicious, ensuring you have the fuel you need to tackle the rest of your day with vitality and joy.

Kale and Quinoa Salad

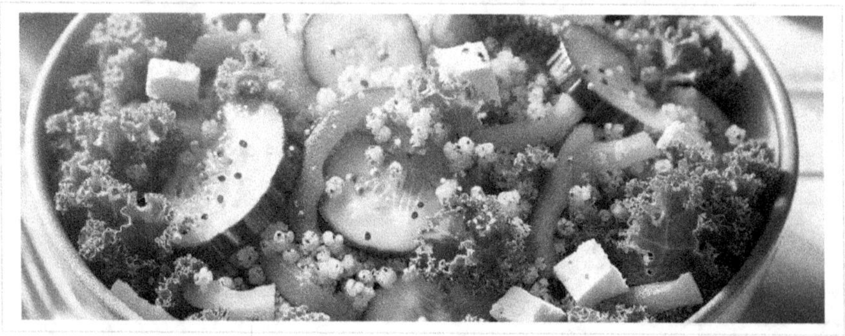

Ingredients:

- 2 cups kale, stems removed and leaves chopped
- 1 cup cooked quinoa
- 1 red bell pepper, thinly sliced
- 1 cucumber, diced
- 1/4 cup feta cheese, crumbled
- For the dressing:
  - 2 tablespoons olive oil
  - 1 tablespoon lemon juice
  - 1 teaspoon honey
  - Salt and pepper to taste

Preparation:

1. In a large bowl, combine the chopped kale, cooked quinoa, sliced red bell pepper, and diced cucumber.
2. In a small bowl, whisk together olive oil, lemon juice, honey, salt, and pepper to create the dressing.
3. Pour the dressing over the salad and toss well to ensure all ingredients are evenly coated.
4. Sprinkle crumbled feta cheese over the top before serving.

Nutritional Values:

- Calories: 280 kcal
- Protein: 9 g
- Carbohydrates: 38 g
- Fat: 12 g
- Fiber: 6 g

Cooking Time: 15 minutes

Serves: 2　　　　　　　　**Rating:** ★★★★★

This Kale and Quinoa Salad is a powerhouse of nutrition and flavor, combining the hearty textures of kale and quinoa with the freshness of vegetables and the tanginess of lemon vinaigrette. It's a perfect, light yet fulfilling meal for any lunchtime.

Turkey Avocado Wraps

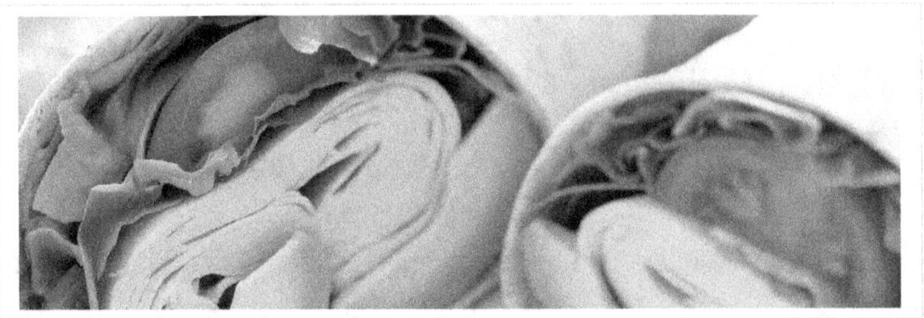

Ingredients:

- 2 whole grain tortillas
- 4 slices of turkey breast
- 1 ripe avocado, sliced
- 1 tomato, sliced
- Lettuce leaves
- Optional: mustard or mayonnaise, salt and pepper to taste

Preparation:

1. Lay out the tortillas on a flat surface.
2. Spread a thin layer of mustard or mayonnaise on each tortilla, if using.
3. Place two slices of turkey breast on each tortilla.

4. Add slices of avocado and tomato, and top with lettuce leaves.

5. Season with salt and pepper to taste.

6. Roll the tortillas tightly, then cut in half to serve.

Nutritional Values:

- Calories: 350 kcal per wrap
- Protein: 25 g
- Carbohydrates: 35 g
- Fat: 15 g
- Fiber: 9 g

Cooking Time: 10 minutes

Serves: 2   **Rating:** ★★★★★

These Turkey Avocado Wraps are the perfect blend of simplicity and flavor, making for a quick, nutritious, and satisfying lunch option. Fresh, creamy avocado and lean turkey wrapped in a whole grain tortilla provide a balanced meal that's both delicious and healthy.

Broccoli and Chickpea Bowl

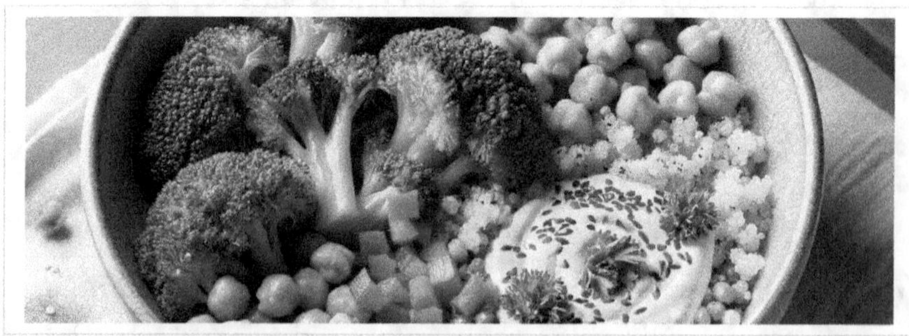

Ingredients:

- 1 cup broccoli florets, roasted
- 1 cup cooked chickpeas
- 1/2 cup cooked quinoa
- 1 red bell pepper, diced
- 2 tablespoons tahini sauce
- Garnish: sesame seeds, fresh parsley

Preparation:

1. Preheat your oven to 400°F (200°C) and roast the broccoli florets with a little olive oil, salt, and pepper until tender and slightly crispy, about 20-25 minutes.
2. In a bowl, layer the cooked quinoa as the base.
3. Add the roasted broccoli, cooked chickpeas, and diced red bell pepper on top of the quinoa.
4. Drizzle tahini sauce over the bowl.
5. Garnish with sesame seeds and fresh parsley.

Nutritional Values:

- Calories: 420 kcal
- Protein: 18 g
- Carbohydrates: 55 g
- Fat: 16 g
- Fiber: 15 g

Cooking Time: 30 minutes

Serves: 2

Rating: ★★★★★

This Broccoli and Chickpea Bowl is a nourishing and flavorful dish, perfect for a wholesome lunch. Packed with protein, fiber, and a variety of nutrients, it's a satisfying meal that supports a healthy lifestyle.

Grilled Chicken Salad

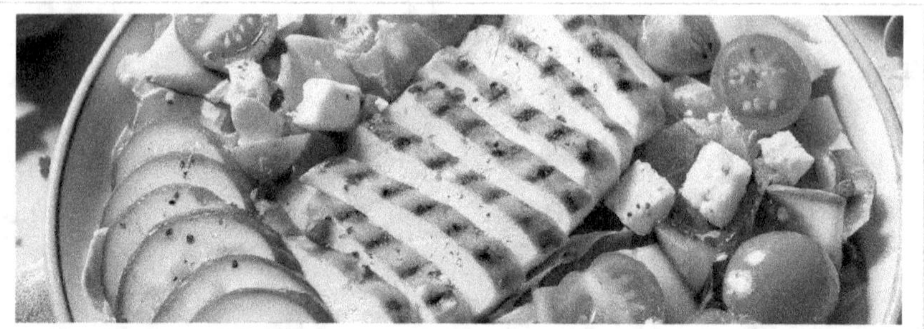

Ingredients:

- 1 grilled chicken breast, sliced
- 2 cups mixed greens
- 1/2 cup cherry tomatoes, halved
- 1/2 cucumber, sliced
- 1 avocado, cut into wedges
- 2 tablespoons feta cheese, crumbled
- 1/4 cup croutons
- Dressing:
  - 2 tablespoons olive oil
  - 1 tablespoon balsamic vinegar
  - Salt and pepper to taste

Preparation:

1. Arrange the mixed greens on a plate as the base.
2. Top with slices of grilled chicken breast, cherry tomatoes, cucumber slices, and avocado wedges.

3. Sprinkle crumbled feta cheese and croutons over the salad.

4. In a small bowl, whisk together olive oil, balsamic vinegar, salt, and pepper to make the dressing.

5. Drizzle the dressing over the salad just before serving.

Nutritional Values:

- Calories: 450 kcal
- Protein: 32 g
- Carbohydrates: 20 g
- Fat: 29 g
- Fiber: 8 g

Cooking Time: 20 minutes

Serves: 2

Rating: ★★★★★

This Grilled Chicken Salad is a perfect balance of flavors and textures, combining lean protein, fresh veggies, and a tangy dressing for a refreshing and satisfying meal.

Butternut Squash Soup

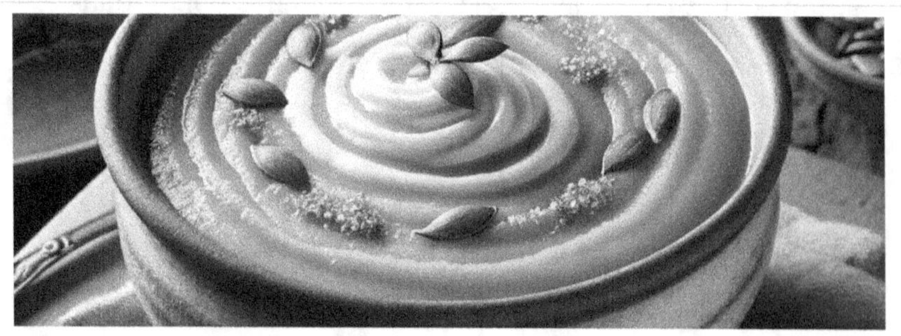

Ingredients:

- 1 medium butternut squash, peeled, seeded, and cubed
- 1 onion, diced
- 2 cloves garlic, minced
- 4 cups vegetable broth
- 1 cup coconut milk
- Salt and pepper to taste
- Olive oil for sautéing
- Optional for garnish: a swirl of cream, roasted pumpkin seeds

Preparation:

1. In a large pot, heat a splash of olive oil over medium heat. Add the diced onion and minced garlic, sautéing until soft and fragrant.

2. Add the cubed butternut squash to the pot, stirring to combine. Cook for a few minutes, then pour in the vegetable broth.

3. Bring to a boil, then reduce heat and simmer until the squash is tender, about 20 minutes.

4. Use an immersion blender to puree the soup until smooth. Stir in the coconut milk, and season with salt and pepper to taste.

5. Serve hot, garnished with a swirl of cream and a sprinkle of roasted pumpkin seeds if desired.

Nutritional Values:

- Calories: 180 kcal per serving
- Protein: 3 g
- Carbohydrates: 27 g
- Fat: 7 g
- Fiber: 5 g

Cooking Time: 35 minutes

Serves: 4   **Rating:** ★★★★★

This Butternut Squash Soup is the essence of comfort food, blending the natural sweetness of squash with the creaminess of coconut milk for a warming, autumnal dish. It's perfect for a cozy meal, delivering both nutrition and satisfying flavors.

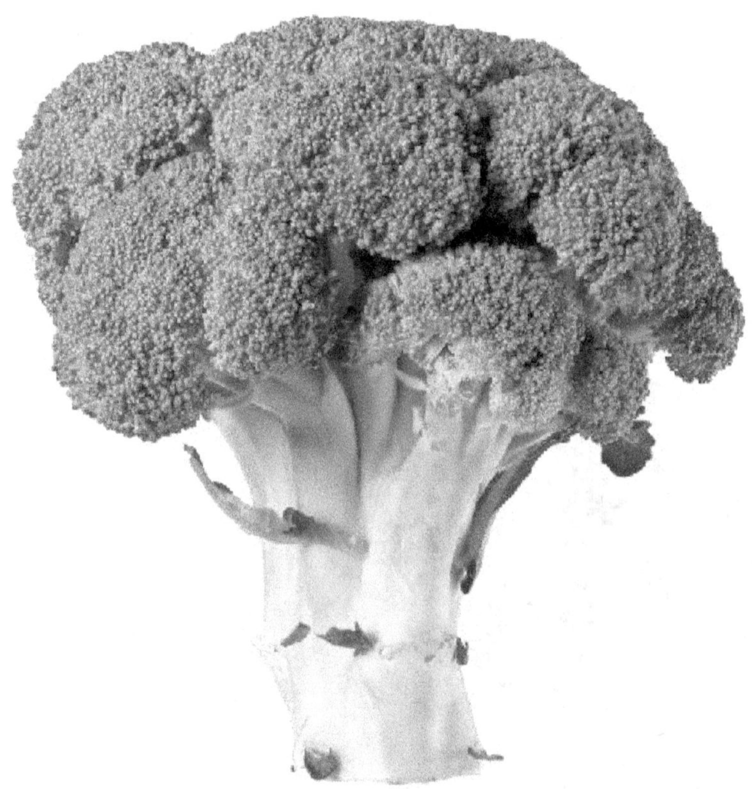

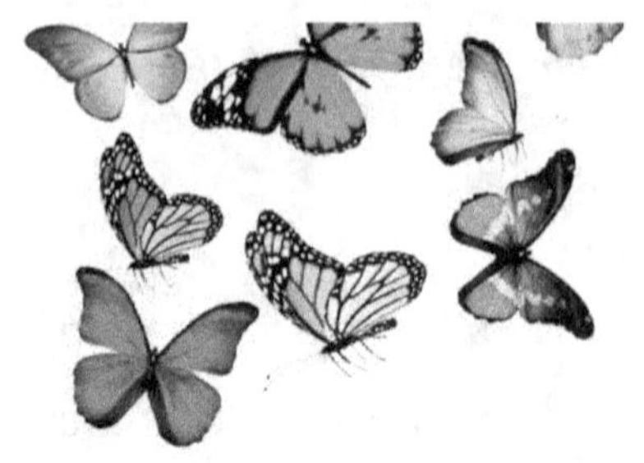

"Nourishing your body with the right foods can turn the tide against Hashimoto's. You're on the right path; every health-conscious decision you make is a powerful stride toward healing."

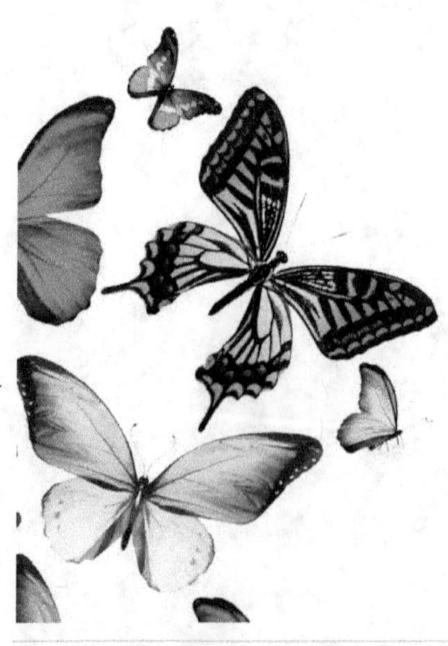

CHAPTER 4: DINNER

Dinner is more than just the last meal of the day; it's an opportunity to unwind, contemplate, and refuel with sustenance and flavors that comfort and satisfy. This section delves into dinners that cater to the needs of persons managing Hashimoto's, with an emphasis on recipes that are both nourishing for the body and delicious for the palate. From the simplicity of grilled salmon with a side of greens to the heartiness of a lentil stew, each food is intended to promote thyroid health while also bringing joy to the dinner table. These meals find a compromise between convenience of preparation and nutritious value, guaranteeing that even on your busiest days, you can enjoy a dinner that feels like a soothing hug for your body.

Grilled Salmon with Asparagus

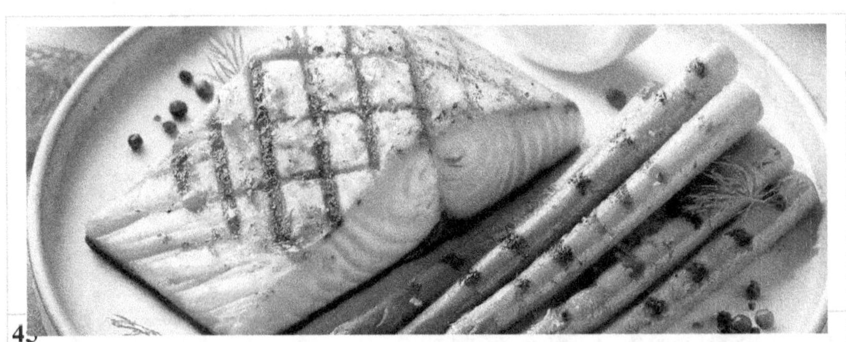

Ingredients:

- 2 salmon fillets (6 oz each)
- 1 lb asparagus, trimmed
- 2 tablespoons olive oil
- Salt and pepper to taste
- Lemon wedges and fresh dill for garnish

Preparation:

1. Preheat your grill to medium-high heat.
2. Brush the salmon fillets and asparagus with olive oil, then season with salt and pepper.
3. Grill the salmon, skin-side down, until cooked through and easily flaked with a fork, about 6-8 minutes per side, depending on thickness.
4. Grill the asparagus alongside the salmon, turning occasionally, until tender and charred, about 5-7 minutes.
5. Serve the grilled salmon and asparagus with lemon wedges and a sprinkle of fresh dill.

Nutritional Values:

- Calories: 400 kcal per serving
- Protein: 34 g
- Carbohydrates: 6 g
- Fat: 28 g
- Fiber: 3 g

Cooking Time: 15 minutes

Serves: 2

Rating: ★★★★★

This Grilled Salmon with Asparagus is a quintessential healthy dinner, offering a perfect balance of lean protein and greens. With the subtle smokiness from the grill and the freshness of lemon and dill, it's a dish that's both simple to prepare and sophisticated in flavor.

Beef Stir-Fry with Broccoli

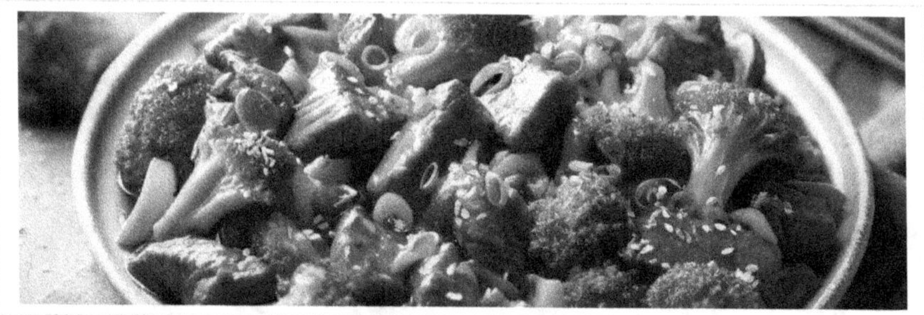

Ingredients:

- 1 lb beef sirloin, thinly sliced
- 2 cups broccoli florets
- 2 tablespoons vegetable oil
- 2 cloves garlic, minced
- 1 tablespoon ginger, minced

- For the sauce:
- 1/4 cup soy sauce
- 2 tablespoons oyster sauce
- 1 tablespoon sesame oil
- 1 teaspoon sugar
- 1/2 cup water
- 1 tablespoon cornstarch

Preparation:

1. In a small bowl, whisk together the soy sauce, oyster sauce, sesame oil, sugar, water, and cornstarch to make the sauce. Set aside.
2. Heat vegetable oil in a large skillet or wok over high heat. Add the beef and stir-fry until browned, about 2-3 minutes. Remove beef from the skillet and set aside.
3. In the same skillet, add a bit more oil if needed, then add the garlic and ginger. Stir-fry for about 30 seconds until fragrant.
4. Add the broccoli and stir-fry for another 3-4 minutes, or until it starts to soften.
5. Return the beef to the skillet. Pour the sauce over the beef and broccoli, stirring well to coat. Cook for another 2-3 minutes, or until the sauce has thickened and the broccoli is tender.
6. Garnish with sesame seeds and green onions before serving.

Nutritional Values:

- Calories: 300 kcal per serving
- Protein: 25 g
- Carbohydrates: 15 g
- Fat: 15 g
- Fiber: 3 g

Cooking Time: 20 minutes

Serves: 4

Rating: ★★★★★

This Beef Stir-Fry with Broccoli is a classic dish that's both flavorful and easy to prepare, making it the perfect choice for a nutritious, satisfying dinner on busy weeknights.

Spaghetti Squash with Marinara Sauce

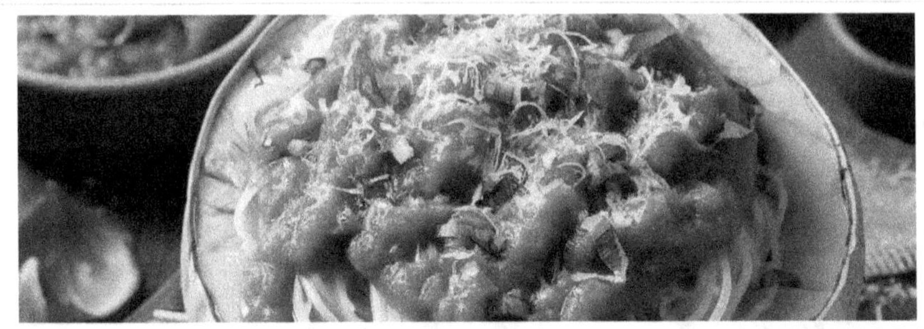

Ingredients:

- 1 medium spaghetti squash
- 2 cups marinara sauce
- 2 tablespoons olive oil
- Salt and pepper to taste
- Fresh basil leaves, for garnish
- Grated Parmesan cheese, for garnish

Preparation:

1. Preheat the oven to 400°F (200°C). Halve the spaghetti squash lengthwise and scoop out the seeds.

2. Brush the inside of each half with olive oil and season with salt and pepper.

3. Place the squash halves cut-side down on a baking sheet and roast until tender, about 40 minutes.

4. Once cool enough to handle, use a fork to scrape the squash into strands, creating "spaghetti."

5. Heat the marinara sauce in a saucepan over medium heat.

6. Top the spaghetti squash strands with warm marinara sauce.

7. Garnish with fresh basil leaves and a sprinkle of grated Parmesan cheese before serving.

Nutritional Values:

- Calories: 180 kcal per serving
- Protein: 4 g
- Carbohydrates: 20 g
- Fat: 10 g
- Fiber: 5 g

Cooking Time: 50 minutes

Serves: 4

Rating: ★★★★★

This Spaghetti Squash with Marinara Sauce offers a delightful, low-carb alternative to traditional pasta dishes.

Chicken and Vegetable Skewers

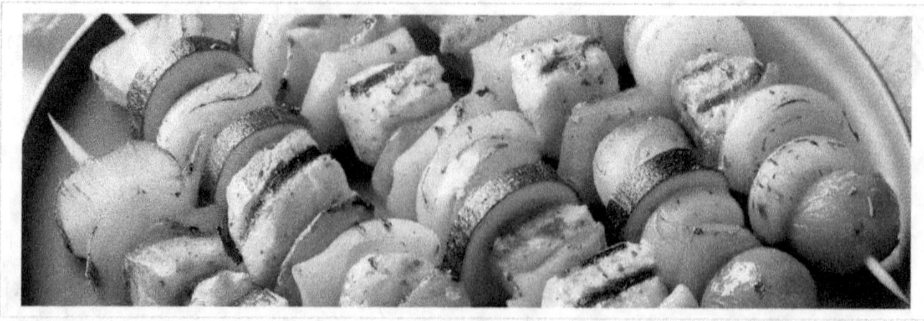

Ingredients:

- 1 lb chicken breast, cut into cubes
- 1 red bell pepper, cut into chunks
- 1 green bell pepper, cut into chunks
- 1 yellow onion, cut into chunks
- 1 zucchini, sliced into rounds
- 2 tablespoons olive oil

- 2 cloves garlic, minced
- 1 teaspoon dried oregano
- Salt and pepper to taste

Marinade:

- 1/4 cup olive oil
- 2 tablespoons lemon juice
- 1 tablespoon balsamic vinegar
- 1 teaspoon honey
- Salt and pepper to taste

Preparation:

1. In a bowl, whisk together the marinade ingredients. Add the chicken cubes and toss to coat. Marinate in the refrigerator for at least 30 minutes, or up to 4 hours.
2. Preheat the grill to medium-high heat.
3. Thread the marinated chicken, bell peppers, onion, and zucchini onto skewers.
4. Brush the skewers with olive oil and season with garlic, oregano, salt, and pepper.
5. Grill the skewers, turning occasionally, until the chicken is cooked through and the vegetables are tender, about 10-15 minutes.

6. Serve hot, optionally with tzatziki sauce or a light salad on the side.

Nutritional Values:

- Calories: 250 kcal per skewer
- Protein: 26 g
- Carbohydrates: 10 g
- Fat: 12 g
- Fiber: 2 g

Cooking Time: 25 minutes (plus marinating time)

Serves: 4

Rating: ★★★★★

These Chicken and Vegetable Skewers offer a delicious way to enjoy a mix of protein and vibrant vegetables, all grilled to bring out their flavors.

Lentil and Sweet Potato Stew

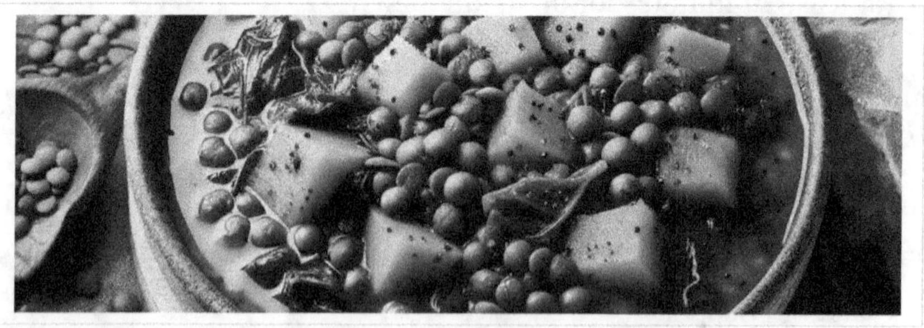

Ingredients:

- 1 cup dried lentils, rinsed
- 1 large sweet potato, peeled and cubed

- 1 onion, diced
- 2 cloves garlic, minced
- 4 cups vegetable broth
- 2 cups water
- 1 teaspoon ground cumin
- 1/2 teaspoon smoked paprika
- Salt and pepper to taste
- 2 cups kale or spinach, chopped
- 1 tablespoon olive oil

Preparation:

1. Heat olive oil in a large pot over medium heat. Add onion and garlic, sautéing until softened.
2. Add the sweet potatoes, lentils, vegetable broth, water, cumin, smoked paprika, salt, and pepper. Bring to a boil, then reduce heat and simmer, covered, until lentils and sweet potatoes are tender, about 25-30 minutes.
3. Stir in the kale or spinach and cook until wilted, about 5 minutes.
4. Adjust seasoning to taste. Serve hot, accompanied by crusty bread for dipping.

Nutritional Values:

- Calories: 300 kcal per serving
- Protein: 18 g
- Carbohydrates: 55 g
- Fat: 3 g
- Fiber: 15 g

Cooking Time: 40 minutes

Serves: 4

Rating: ★★★★★

This Lentil and Sweet Potato Stew is a comforting and nutritious meal, perfect for chilly evenings. It combines hearty lentils and sweet potatoes with the warmth of spices and the nourishing goodness of greens for a wholesome dish that's both satisfying and healthy.

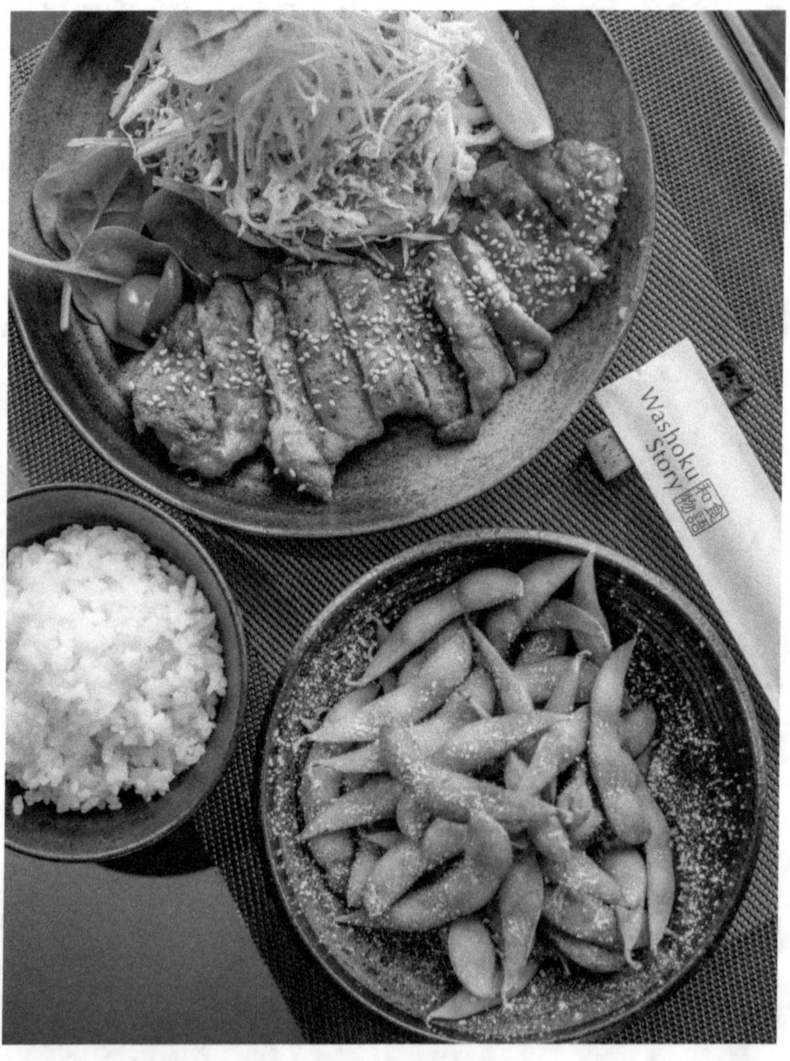

CHAPTER 5: SALADS

In the Salads section, we celebrate the vivid world of fresh, nutrient-dense foods that combine to produce healthful and tasty dishes. Here, you'll find a wide variety of salads, from leafy greens decked with colorful vegetables, fruits, nuts, and seeds to hearty grain-based salads that promise to satisfy. Each recipe is deliberately crafted not just to satisfy your taste senses but also to benefit your health, which is especially good for persons with Hashimoto's. Whether you're looking for a light and refreshing side dish or a filling meal, these salads are a great way to get a variety of nutrients into your diet while keeping your meals interesting and enjoyable. Let's dig into the freshness and discover salads that may stand alone as a meal or add flavor and texture to any dish.

Arugula and Beet Salad

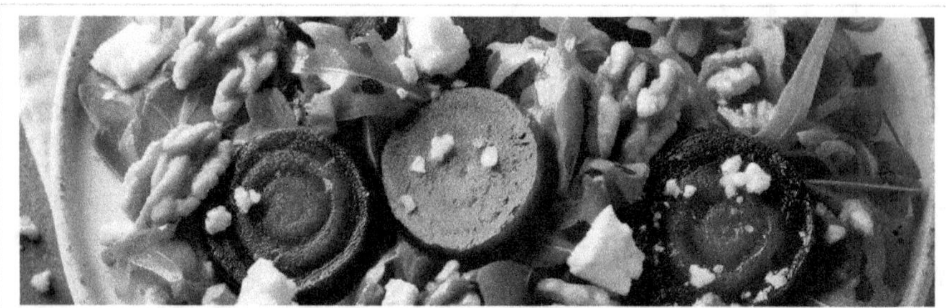

Ingredients:

- 4 cups arugula leaves
- 2 medium beets, roasted and sliced
- 1/2 cup crumbled goat cheese
- 1/4 cup toasted walnuts
- Dressing:
- 2 tablespoons balsamic vinegar
- 4 tablespoons olive oil
- 1 teaspoon honey
- Salt and pepper to taste

Preparation:

1. To prepare the dressing, whisk together balsamic vinegar, olive oil, honey, salt, and pepper in a small bowl until well combined.
2. In a large salad bowl, toss the arugula leaves with the dressing until evenly coated.
3. Top the dressed arugula with sliced roasted beets, crumbled goat cheese, and toasted walnuts.
4. Serve immediately, ensuring the fresh flavors and textures remain at their peak.

Nutritional Values:

- Calories: 250 kcal per serving
- Protein: 8 g
- Carbohydrates: 12 g
- Fat: 20 g
- Fiber: 3 g

Cooking Time: 10 minutes (excluding time to roast beets)

Serves: 4   **Rating:** ★★★★★

This Arugula and Beet Salad is a celebration of flavors and textures, combining the peppery bite of arugula with the earthy sweetness of beets, the creamy tang of goat cheese, and the crunch of walnuts. Drizzled with a honey-balsamic vinaigrette, it's a sophisticated salad that's perfect for any occasion.

Carrot and Cabbage Slaw

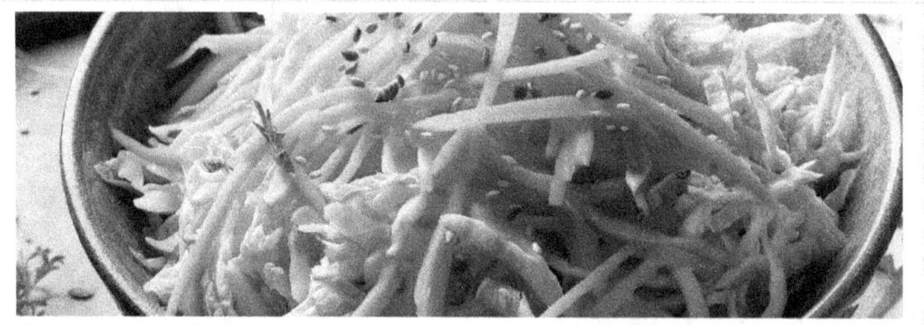

Ingredients:

- 2 cups green cabbage, finely shredded
- 1 cup carrots, grated
- 2 tablespoons olive oil
- 1 tablespoon apple cider vinegar
- 1 teaspoon honey
- Salt and pepper to taste
- Optional garnishes: sesame seeds, fresh parsley or cilantro

Preparation:

1. In a large mixing bowl, combine the shredded cabbage and grated carrots.

2. In a small bowl, whisk together olive oil, apple cider vinegar, honey, salt, and pepper to create the dressing.

3. Pour the dressing over the cabbage and carrot mixture, tossing until well coated.

4. Refrigerate for at least 30 minutes to allow the flavors to meld.

5. Before serving, sprinkle with sesame seeds and fresh herbs for an extra touch of flavor and texture.

Nutritional Values:

- Calories: 120 kcal per serving
- Protein: 1 g
- Carbohydrates: 10 g
- Fat: 9 g
- Fiber: 2 g

Cooking Time: 10 minutes + chilling time

Serves: 4　　　　　　　　**Rating:** ★★★★★

This Carrot and Cabbage Slaw is a crisp, vibrant, and refreshing side dish that pairs beautifully with a variety of mains.

Cucumber and Tomato Salad

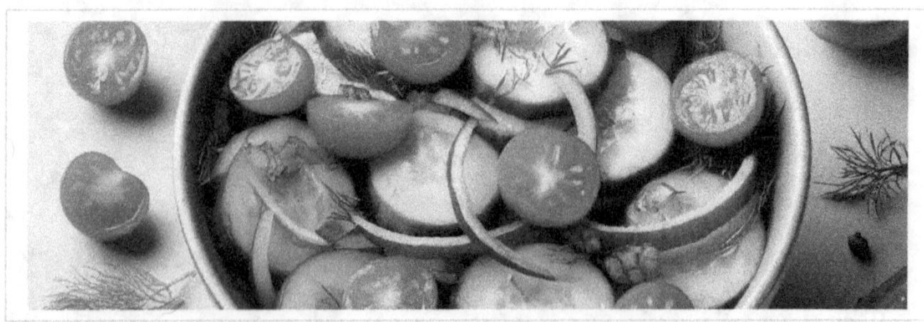

Ingredients:

- 2 large cucumbers, sliced
- 2 cups cherry tomatoes, halved
- 1/2 red onion, thinly sliced
- 3 tablespoons olive oil
- 1 tablespoon vinegar (white or apple cider)
- Salt and pepper to taste
- Fresh dill or parsley, chopped (for garnish)

Preparation:

1. In a large salad bowl, combine the sliced cucumbers, halved cherry tomatoes, and thinly sliced red onion.
2. Drizzle with olive oil and vinegar. Toss gently to coat all the vegetables evenly.
3. Season with salt and pepper according to taste.
4. Garnish with chopped fresh dill or parsley for a burst of flavor and a touch of color.
5. Serve immediately or let it chill in the refrigerator for about 30 minutes before serving to enhance the flavors.

Nutritional Values:

- Calories: 100 kcal per serving
- Protein: 2 g
- Carbohydrates: 8 g
- Fat: 7 g
- Fiber: 2 g

Cooking Time: 10 minutes

Serves: 4   **Rating:** ★★★★★

This Cucumber and Tomato Salad is the epitome of a refreshing side dish, perfect for hot summer days or as a light addition to any meal. Its crisp textures and bright flavors are sure to delight your taste buds.

Spinach and Strawberry Salad

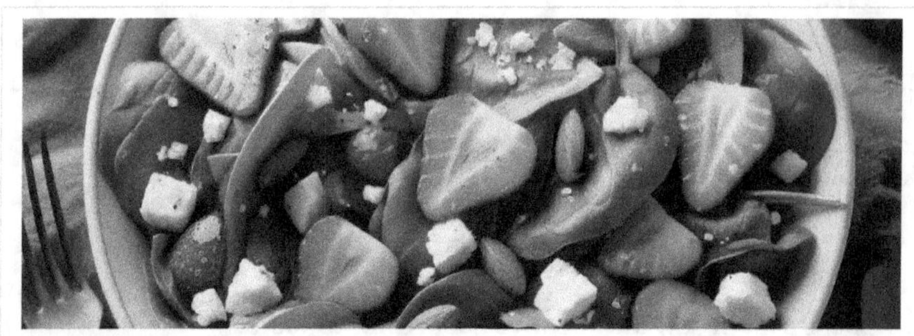

Ingredients:

- 4 cups fresh spinach leaves
- 1 cup strawberries, sliced
- 1/4 cup slivered almonds
- 1/2 cup crumbled feta cheese
- Dressing:
- 2 tablespoons balsamic vinegar
- 1 tablespoon olive oil
- 1 teaspoon honey
- Salt and pepper to taste

Preparation:

1. In a large salad bowl, combine the spinach leaves and sliced strawberries.

2. Toast the slivered almonds in a dry pan over medium heat until golden and fragrant, then sprinkle over the salad.

3. Add the crumbled feta cheese to the bowl.

4. In a small bowl, whisk together the balsamic vinegar, olive oil, honey, salt, and pepper to make the dressing.

5. Drizzle the dressing over the salad and toss gently to combine.

6. Serve immediately to ensure the spinach stays fresh and the strawberries maintain their vibrant color.

Nutritional Values:

- Calories: 180 kcal per serving
- Protein: 6 g
- Carbohydrates: 10 g
- Fat: 13 g
- Fiber: 3 g

Cooking Time: 10 minutes

Serves: 4   **Rating:** ★★★★★

This Spinach and Strawberry Salad is a harmonious blend of sweet and savory, combining the earthiness of spinach with the sweetness of strawberries, the crunch of almonds, and the creaminess of feta, all tied together with a tangy balsamic dressing. It's a refreshing, nutritious dish perfect for any occasion.

Mixed Greens with Avocado

Ingredients:

- 4 cups mixed greens (arugula, spinach, lettuce)
- 1 ripe avocado, sliced
- 2 tablespoons sunflower seeds
- 1/4 cup crumbled goat cheese
- Dressing:
  - 3 tablespoons olive oil
  - 1 tablespoon lemon juice
  - Salt and pepper to taste

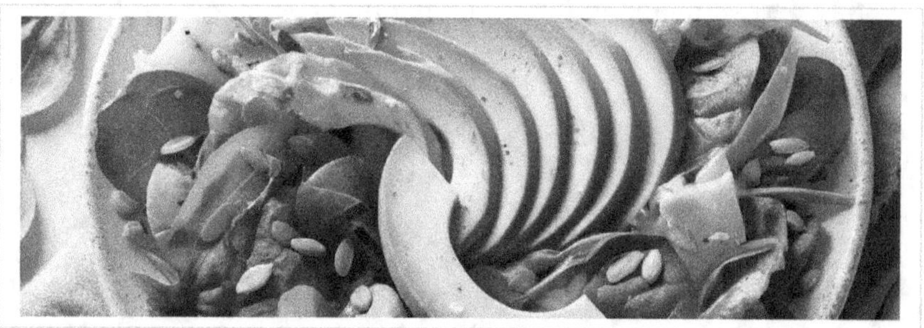

Preparation:

1. In a large salad bowl, combine the mixed greens and sliced avocado.
2. In a small bowl, whisk together olive oil, lemon juice, salt, and pepper to make the dressing.
3. Drizzle the dressing over the salad and toss gently to coat.
4. Sprinkle sunflower seeds and crumbled goat cheese over the top.
5. Serve immediately, enjoying the contrast between the creamy avocado and the crisp greens.

Nutritional Values:

- Calories: 220 kcal per serving
- Protein: 6 g
- Carbohydrates: 10 g
- Fat: 19 g
- Fiber: 7 g

Cooking Time: 10 minutes

Serves: 4

Rating: ★★★★★

This Mixed Greens with Avocado Salad is a testament to simplicity and nutrition, blending the lush textures and flavors of fresh greens with the richness of avocado. It's a versatile dish that serves as a perfect side or a light, healthy meal on its own.

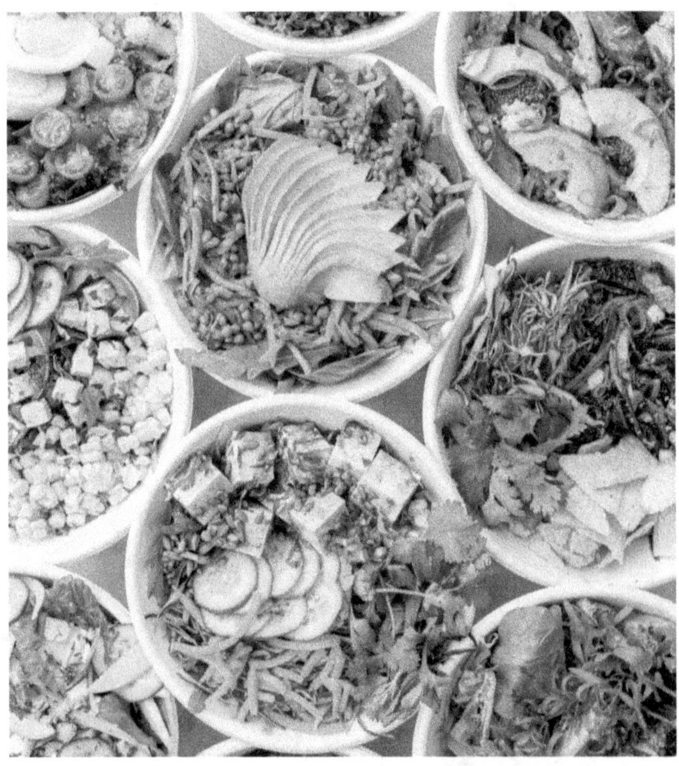

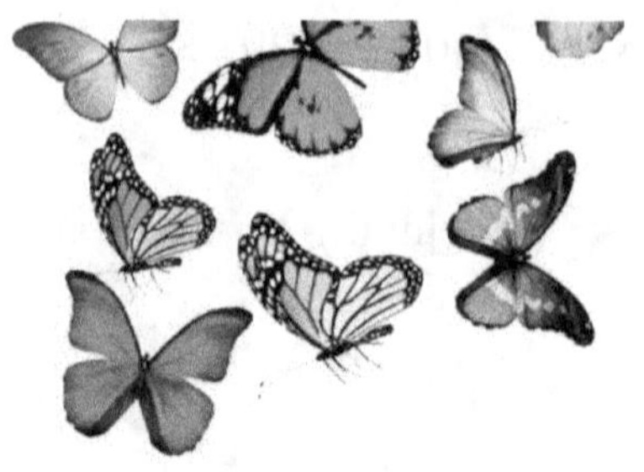

"Remember, healing starts on your plate. Choose foods that loves you back, those that bring not only pleasure but also healing and strength to your body."

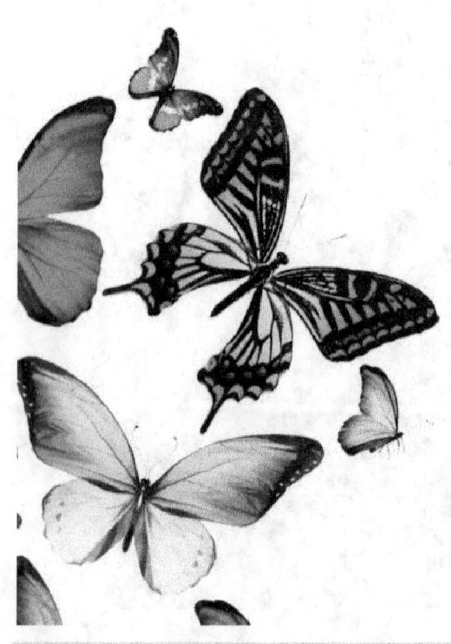

CHAPTER 6: STEW

These recipes have been painstakingly designed to promote wellness, especially for people dealing with Hashimoto's disease. Each stew blends a rich tapestry of ingredients that are cooked to perfection, resulting in meals that are both restorative and tasty. From the sturdiness of a classic beef stew to the delicate aromas of a vegetable medley, these recipes are intended to be both accessible and genuinely fulfilling. Whether you like the simplicity of a one-pot meal or the slow-cooked intricacy of layered tastes, our stew recipes are sure to offer warmth, comfort, and nourishment to your table. Let's enjoy the soothing power of a wonderful stew, where each mouthful brings us closer to feeling our best.

Moroccan Chickpea Stew

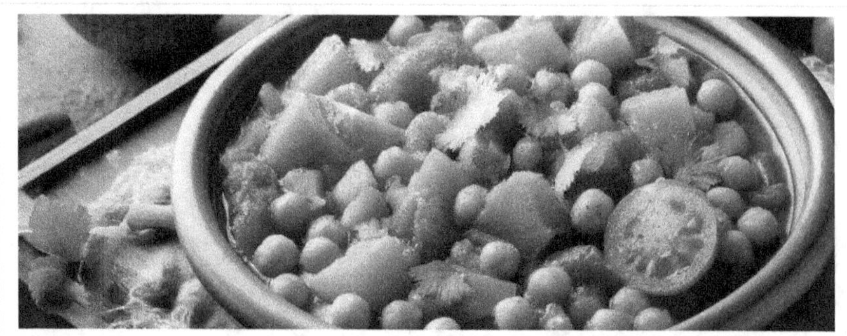

Ingredients:

- 2 cans chickpeas, drained and rinsed
- 1 large sweet potato, cubed
- 2 carrots, sliced
- 1 onion, diced
- 3 cloves garlic, minced
- 1 can diced tomatoes
- 4 cups vegetable broth
- 2 teaspoons ground cumin
- 1 teaspoon ground coriander
- 1/2 teaspoon ground cinnamon
- 1/2 teaspoon cayenne pepper (adjust to taste)
- Salt and pepper to taste
- 2 tablespoons olive oil
- Fresh cilantro or parsley, for garnish

Preparation:

1. Heat olive oil in a large pot over medium heat. Add onion and garlic, cooking until softened.
2. Stir in the spices (cumin, coriander, cinnamon, cayenne pepper, salt, and pepper), and cook for another minute until fragrant.
3. Add the chickpeas, sweet potato, carrots, diced tomatoes, and vegetable broth. Bring to a boil, then reduce heat to simmer.
4. Cover and cook for about 25-30 minutes, or until the sweet potatoes and carrots are tender.
5. Serve hot, garnished with fresh cilantro or parsley.

Nutritional Values:

- Calories: 260 kcal per serving
- Protein: 9 g
- Carbohydrates: 45 g
- Fat: 6 g
- Fiber: 12 g

Cooking Time: 40 minutes

Serves: 4

Rating: ★★★★★

This Moroccan Chickpea Stew is a celebration of flavors and textures, combining hearty chickpeas with sweet potatoes and spices for a comforting and nutritious meal. Perfect for a cozy dinner, it's a dish that brings the essence of Moroccan cuisine right to your table.

Beef and Vegetable Stew

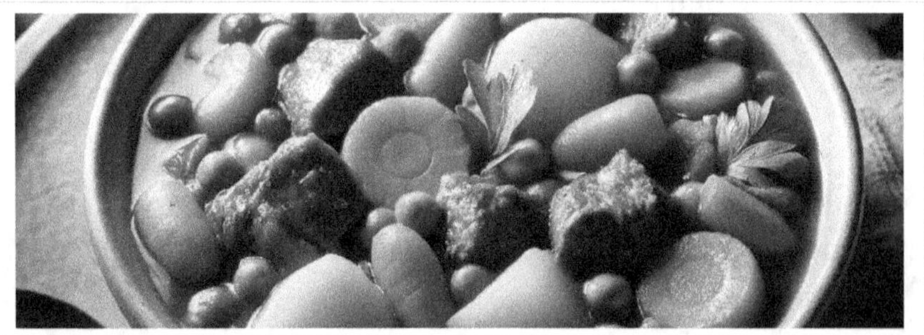

Ingredients:

- 1 lb beef stew meat, cut into chunks
- 2 carrots, peeled and sliced
- 2 potatoes, peeled and cubed
- 1 cup peas
- 1 onion, chopped

- 2 cloves garlic, minced
- 4 cups beef broth
- 1 tablespoon tomato paste
- 2 tablespoons flour
- 2 tablespoons olive oil
- Salt and pepper to taste
- Fresh parsley, chopped for garnish

Preparation:

1. In a large pot, heat olive oil over medium-high heat. Season the beef with salt and pepper, then brown in batches, setting aside once done.
2. In the same pot, add the onion and garlic, cooking until softened.
3. Sprinkle flour over the onions and garlic, cooking for a minute before stirring in the tomato paste.
4. Gradually add the beef broth, scraping up any browned bits from the bottom of the pot.
5. Return the beef to the pot along with carrots and potatoes. Bring to a boil, then reduce to a simmer, covering and cooking until the beef is tender, about 1.5 to 2 hours.
6. Add the peas during the last 10 minutes of cooking.
7. Adjust seasoning with salt and pepper. Garnish with fresh parsley before serving.

Nutritional Values:

- Calories: 350 kcal per serving
- Protein: 35 g
- Carbohydrates: 25 g
- Fat: 12 g
- Fiber: 5 g

Cooking Time: 2 hours 20 minutes

Serves: 4   **Rating:** ★★★★★

This Beef and Vegetable Stew is a quintessential comfort food, offering a rich blend of tender beef, hearty vegetables, and a flavorful broth. It's a filling, nutritious meal perfect for chilly evenings or any time you need a warm, comforting dish.

Chicken and Kale Stew

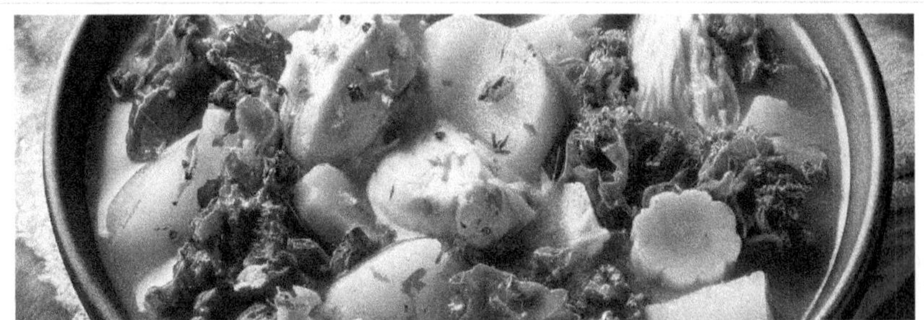

Ingredients:

- 1 lb chicken breasts, cut into chunks
- 4 cups chopped kale
- 2 carrots, sliced
- 2 potatoes, cubed
- 1 onion, diced
- 2 cloves garlic, minced
- 4 cups chicken broth
- 1 teaspoon thyme
- Salt and pepper to taste
- 2 tablespoons olive oil

Preparation:

1. Heat olive oil in a large pot over medium heat. Add the chicken pieces, season with salt and pepper, and cook until browned. Remove chicken and set aside.

2. In the same pot, add the onion and garlic, sautéing until soft.

3. Add the carrots and potatoes, cooking for a few minutes before returning the chicken to the pot.

4. Pour in the chicken broth, add thyme, and bring to a boil. Reduce heat, cover, and simmer for about 20 minutes, or until vegetables are tender.

5. Add the kale in the last 5 minutes of cooking, allowing it to wilt.

6. Adjust seasoning with salt and pepper. Serve hot.

Nutritional Values:

- Calories: 300 kcal per serving
- Protein: 28 g
- Carbohydrates: 22 g
- Fat: 10 g
- Fiber: 5 g

Cooking Time: 35 minutes

Serves: 4

Rating: ★★★★★

This Chicken and Kale Stew is a comforting and nutritious dish, perfect for those chilly days when you crave something warming and hearty. Packed with lean protein, leafy greens, and root vegetables, it's a balanced meal that satisfies both taste and health.

Pumpkin and Lentil Stew

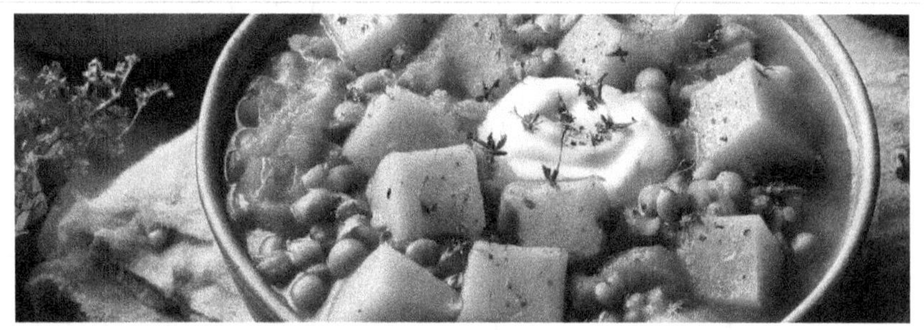

Ingredients:

- 1 lb pumpkin, peeled and cubed
- 1 cup dried lentils, rinsed
- 1 large carrot, diced
- 1 onion, diced
- 2 cloves garlic, minced
- 1 can (14 oz) diced tomatoes
- 4 cups vegetable broth
- 1 teaspoon ground cumin
- 1/2 teaspoon ground cinnamon
- Salt and pepper to taste
- 2 tablespoons olive oil
- Optional for garnish: dollop of yogurt, fresh cilantro or parsley

Preparation:

1. Heat olive oil in a large pot over medium heat. Add the onion and garlic, sautéing until soft and fragrant.
2. Add the pumpkin and carrot, cooking for a few minutes until they start to soften.
3. Stir in the lentils, diced tomatoes, vegetable broth, cumin, cinnamon, salt, and pepper.

4. Bring to a boil, then reduce heat and simmer, covered, for about 25-30 minutes, or until the lentils and pumpkin are tender.

5. Taste and adjust seasoning as needed. Serve hot, garnished with a dollop of yogurt and fresh herbs if desired.

Nutritional Values:

- Calories: 250 kcal per serving
- Protein: 10 g
- Carbohydrates: 45 g
- Fat: 4 g
- Fiber: 12 g

Cooking Time: 40 minutes

Serves: 4

Rating: ★★★★★

This Pumpkin and Lentil Stew is a heartwarming dish that combines the sweetness of pumpkin with the earthiness of lentils, spiced with cumin and cinnamon for an autumnal flavor profile.

Seafood Stew

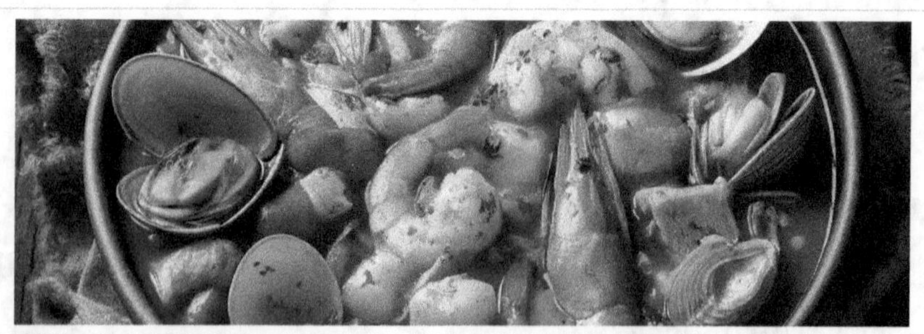

Ingredients:

- 1/2 lb shrimp, peeled and deveined
- 1/2 lb scallops
- 1/2 lb clams, cleaned
- 1/2 lb firm fish fillets (such as cod or halibut), cut into chunks
- 1 onion, diced
- 2 cloves garlic, minced
- 1 can (14 oz) diced tomatoes
- 4 cups fish or vegetable broth
- 1/2 cup white wine (optional)
- 2 tablespoons olive oil
- 1 teaspoon paprika
- Salt and pepper to taste
- Fresh parsley, chopped for garnish
- Crusty bread, for serving

Preparation:

1. Heat olive oil in a large pot over medium heat. Add onion and garlic, sautéing until soft.
2. Pour in the white wine (if using), allowing it to reduce slightly, then add diced tomatoes, fish broth, paprika, salt, and pepper. Bring to a simmer.
3. Add the clams to the pot, cover, and cook until they start to open, about 5 minutes.
4. Add the shrimp, scallops, and fish chunks, simmering until they are cooked through, about 5-7 minutes.
5. Adjust seasoning to taste. Serve the stew in bowls, garnished with fresh parsley.
6. Serve with slices of crusty bread for dipping into the broth.

Nutritional Values:

- Calories: 300 kcal per serving
- Protein: 35 g
- Carbohydrates: 15 g
- Fat: 10 g
- Fiber: 2 g

Cooking Time: 30 minutes

Serves: 4

Rating: ★★★★★

This Seafood Stew is a feast for the senses, brimming with a variety of seafood simmered in a flavorful tomato-based broth. It's a dish that celebrates the bounty of the ocean, offering a luxurious yet comforting meal that's perfect for sharing.

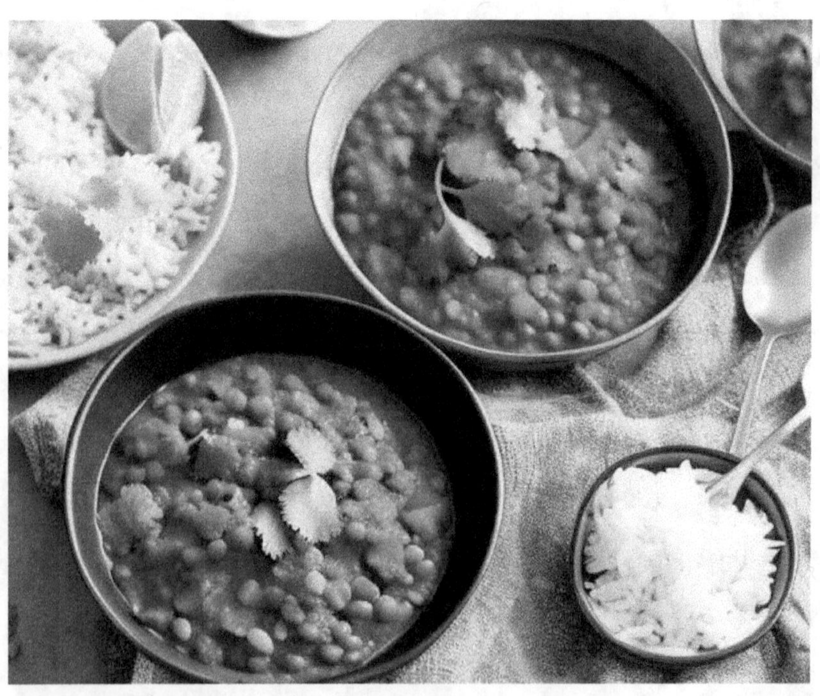

CHAPTER 7: SIDES

These recipes range from simple roasted vegetables and fluffy grains to more elaborate preparations that bring new flavors and textures to the table. Each side dish has been selected not only for its delicious taste but also for its nutritional benefits, ensuring that every meal is as healthy as it is satisfying. Whether you're looking for a quick weeknight addition or something special to impress your guests, you'll find the perfect accompaniment to complete any meal. Dive into these side dishes to discover new favorites that will elevate your dining experience, making every meal more memorable.

Roasted Brussels Sprouts

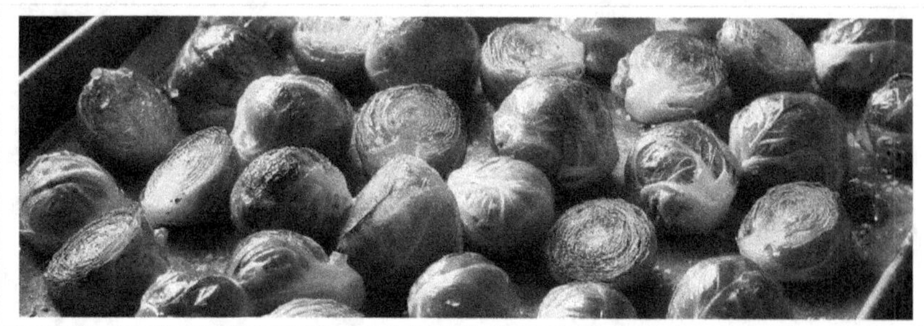

Ingredients:

- 1 lb Brussels sprouts, trimmed and halved
- 2 tablespoons olive oil
- Coarse sea salt, to taste
- Black pepper, to taste

Preparation:

1. Preheat the oven to 400°F (200°C).
2. Toss the Brussels sprouts with olive oil, salt, and pepper until they are well coated.
3. Spread them out in a single layer on a baking sheet.
4. Roast in the oven until they are golden brown and crispy on the outside, about 20-25 minutes, turning halfway through the cooking time.
5. Serve hot, directly from the oven.

Nutritional Values:

- Calories: 80 kcal per serving
- Protein: 3 g
- Carbohydrates: 10 g
- Fat: 4 g
- Fiber: 4 g

Cooking Time: 30 minutes

Serves: 4

Rating: ★★★★★

Roasted Brussels Sprouts transform these humble vegetables into a crispy, golden delight. This simple side dish, with its nutty and slightly sweet flavor, is a testament to the power of roasting, making it a favorite for any meal.

Cauliflower Rice

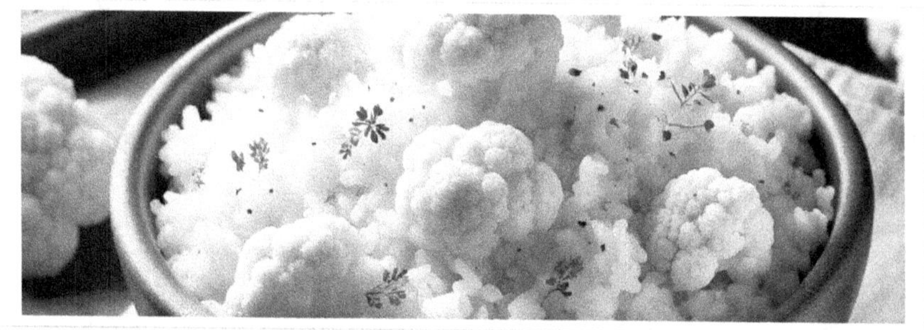

Ingredients:

- 1 large head of cauliflower, cut into florets
- 1 tablespoon olive oil
- Salt and pepper to taste
- Optional: Fresh herbs for garnish (parsley, cilantro, or chives)

Preparation:

1. Wash and thoroughly dry cauliflower florets. Pulse in a food processor until the texture resembles rice grains.
2. Heat olive oil in a large skillet over medium heat. Add the cauliflower rice, salt, and pepper.
3. Cook, stirring occasionally, until the cauliflower is heated through and slightly crispy, about 5-7 minutes.
4. Garnish with fresh herbs if desired before serving.

Nutritional Values:

- Calories: 60 kcal per serving
- Protein: 2 g
- Carbohydrates: 8 g
- Fat: 3 g
- Fiber: 4 g

Cooking Time: 15 minutes

Serves: 4

Rating: ★★★★★

Cauliflower Rice offers a fantastic, low-carb alternative to traditional rice, with a versatile flavor that pairs well with a variety of dishes. Light and fluffy, it's a simple yet delicious side that adds a healthy twist to any meal.

Sautéed Green Beans

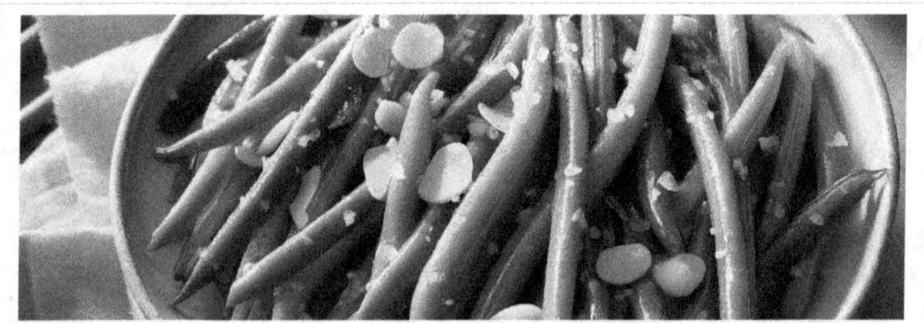

Ingredients:

- 1 lb fresh green beans, trimmed
- 2 tablespoons olive oil
- 2 cloves garlic, minced
- Salt and pepper to taste
- Optional garnishes: slivered almonds, lemon zest

Preparation:

1. Heat olive oil in a large skillet over medium heat.

2. Add the minced garlic and sauté for about 30 seconds, until fragrant.

3. Add the green beans to the skillet, tossing to coat with the olive oil and garlic. Season with salt and pepper.

4. Cook, stirring occasionally, until the beans are tender-crisp, about 5-7 minutes.

5. Transfer to a serving dish and garnish with slivered almonds and lemon zest if desired.

Nutritional Values:

- Calories: 80 kcal per serving
- Protein: 2 g
- Carbohydrates: 8 g
- Fat: 5 g
- Fiber: 4 g

Cooking Time: 12 minutes

Serves: 4

Rating: ★★★★★

Sautéed Green Beans are a delightful side dish, offering a combination of tender-crisp texture and fresh flavors enhanced by garlic. This simple preparation highlights the natural beauty and taste of green beans, making them a versatile addition to any meal.

Mashed Sweet Potatoes

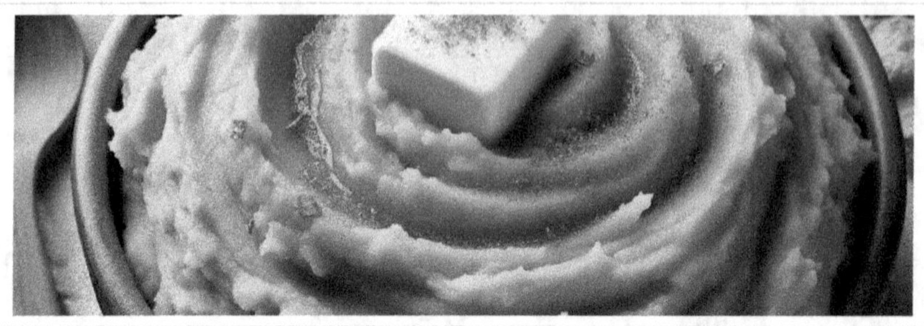

Ingredients:

- 2 lbs sweet potatoes, peeled and cubed
- 4 tablespoons unsalted butter
- 1/4 cup milk or cream
- Salt to taste
- Optional: cinnamon or nutmeg for garnish

Preparation:

1. Place the sweet potato cubes in a large pot and cover with water. Bring to a boil over high heat, then reduce to a simmer and cook until the potatoes are tender, about 15-20 minutes.
2. Drain the sweet potatoes and return them to the pot. Add the butter and milk or cream. Mash until smooth and creamy.
3. Season with salt to taste. For added flavor, sprinkle with cinnamon or nutmeg.
4. Serve warm, with an extra pat of butter on top if desired.

Nutritional Values:

- Calories: 200 kcal per serving
- Protein: 2 g
- Carbohydrates: 35 g
- Fat: 6 g
- Fiber: 5 g

Cooking Time: 25 minutes

Serves: 4

Rating: ★★★★★

Mashed Sweet Potatoes offer a delicious twist on a classic side dish, bringing a natural sweetness and creamy texture to your meal

Zucchini Noodles

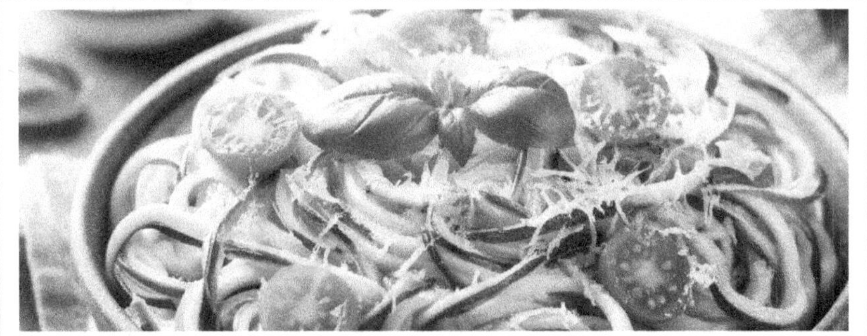

Ingredients:

- 4 medium zucchinis
- 1 tablespoon olive oil
- Salt and pepper to taste
- Optional garnishes: cherry tomatoes, fresh basil, Parmesan cheese shavings

Preparation:

1. Use a spiralizer to turn the zucchinis into noodles. If you don't have a spiralizer, a vegetable peeler can work to create wider noodles.
2. Heat olive oil in a large pan over medium heat. Add the zucchini noodles, seasoning with salt and pepper.
3. Sauté the noodles for 2-3 minutes, just until tender. Be careful not to overcook to keep them al dente.
4. Remove from heat and if desired, toss with garnishes like halved cherry tomatoes, fresh basil, and Parmesan cheese shavings for extra flavor and texture.
5. Serve immediately as a light and healthy alternative to traditional pasta dishes.

Nutritional Values:

- Calories: 70 kcal per serving
- Protein: 2 g
- Carbohydrates: 4 g
- Fat: 5 g
- Fiber: 1 g

Cooking Time: 5 minutes

Serves: 4

Rating: ★★★★★

Zucchini Noodles, or "zoodles," offer a fresh, light, and nutritious option for those looking to enjoy the satisfaction of a pasta dish without the carbs. They're versatile, quick to prepare, and can be paired with a variety of sauces and toppings for a delicious meal.

CHAPTER 8: SEAFOOD AND FISH

Here, you'll discover a treasure trove of recipes that highlight the delicate and diverse tastes of the sea. From the briny sweetness of scallops and the robust flavors of salmon to the light and flaky textures of white fish, each dish is designed to celebrate the natural bounty of the ocean. Whether you're seeking simple, grilled preparations that let the seafood shine or more elaborate dishes with complex sauces and seasonings, this collection offers something for every palate. Embrace the health benefits of a diet rich in omega-3 fatty acids and lean protein with these carefully curated seafood and fish recipes, perfect for elegant dinners, casual gatherings, or nourishing family meals.

Baked Cod with Lemon and Dill

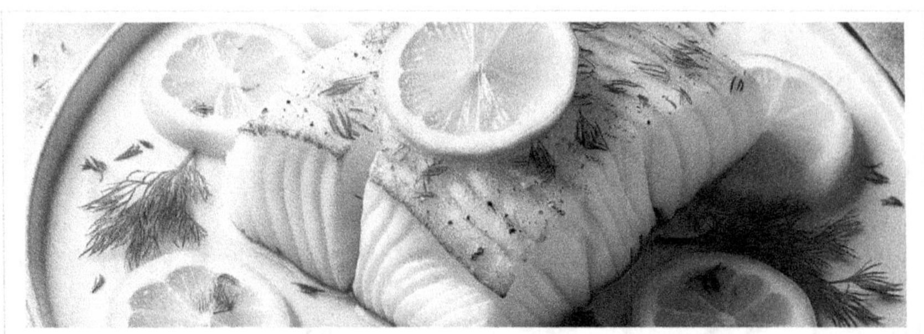

Ingredients:

- 4 cod fillets (6 oz each)
- 2 tablespoons olive oil
- 1 lemon, thinly sliced
- 2 tablespoons fresh dill, chopped
- Salt and pepper to taste

Preparation:

1. Preheat your oven to 400°F (200°C). Lightly grease a baking dish with olive oil.
2. Place cod fillets in the baking dish. Season each fillet with salt and pepper, then drizzle with olive oil.
3. Top each fillet with lemon slices and sprinkle with chopped dill.
4. Bake in the preheated oven until the fish is opaque and flakes easily with a fork, about 12-15 minutes.
5. Serve immediately, garnished with additional lemon slices and dill if desired.

Nutritional Values:

- Calories: 190 kcal per serving
- Protein: 30 g
- Carbohydrates: 2 g
- Fat: 7 g
- Fiber: 0 g

Cooking Time: 15 minutes

Serves: 4

Rating: ★★★★★

Baked Cod with Lemon and Dill is a simple, elegant dish that celebrates the natural flavors of the sea. The bright, citrusy notes of lemon and the subtle hint of dill perfectly complement the tender, flaky texture of the cod, making this a light yet satisfying meal for any occasion.

Shrimp and Avocado Salad

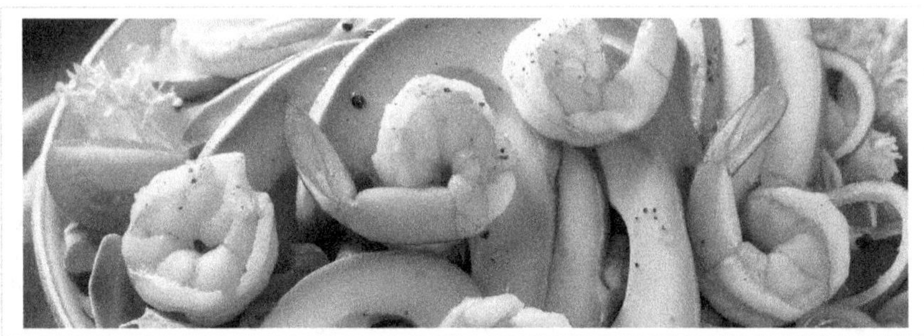

Ingredients:

- 1 lb cooked shrimp, peeled and deveined
- 2 ripe avocados, sliced
- 4 cups mixed greens
- 1 cup cherry tomatoes, halved
- 1/2 cucumber, sliced
- 1/4 red onion, thinly sliced

- Dressing:
  - 3 tablespoons olive oil
  - 1 tablespoon lime juice
  - 1 teaspoon honey
  - Salt and pepper to taste

Preparation:

1. In a large salad bowl, combine mixed greens, cherry tomatoes, cucumber slices, and red onion.
2. Top the salad with cooked shrimp and avocado slices.
3. In a small bowl, whisk together olive oil, lime juice, honey, salt, and pepper to make the dressing.
4. Drizzle the dressing over the salad and gently toss to combine.
5. Serve immediately, enjoying the refreshing blend of flavors.

Nutritional Values:

- Calories: 300 kcal per serving
- Protein: 25 g
- Carbohydrates: 12 g
- Fat: 18 g
- Fiber: 7 g

Cooking Time: 15 minutes

Serves: 4

Rating: ★★★★★

This Shrimp and Avocado Salad is a delightful combination of fresh, crisp vegetables, creamy avocado, and succulent shrimp, all brought together with a zesty lime dressing.

Grilled Tuna Steaks

Ingredients:

- 4 tuna steaks (about 6 oz each)
- 2 tablespoons olive oil
- Salt and pepper to taste
- For the side:

- 1 lb asparagus, trimmed
- 1 bell pepper, sliced
- Garnish:
- Lemon wedges
- Fresh herbs (e.g., parsley or cilantro)

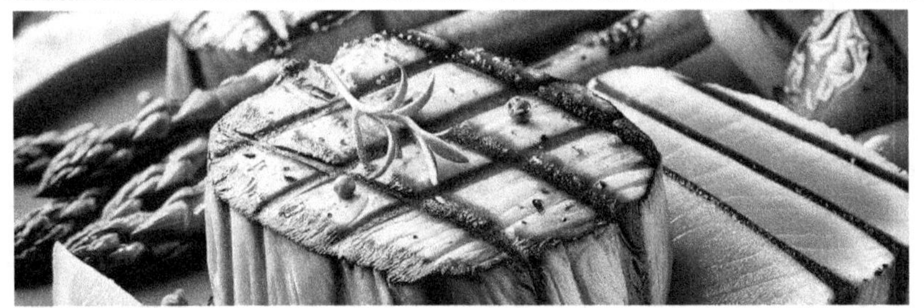

Preparation:

1. Preheat your grill to high heat. Brush both sides of the tuna steaks with olive oil and season with salt and pepper.
2. Grill the tuna steaks for about 2-3 minutes per side for medium-rare, or until desired doneness is reached.
3. In a separate grill pan or basket, grill the asparagus and bell pepper slices, tossing with olive oil, salt, and pepper, until they are tender and slightly charred, about 5-7 minutes.
4. Serve the grilled tuna steaks with the grilled vegetables on the side.
5. Garnish with lemon wedges and a sprinkle of fresh herbs.

Nutritional Values:

- Calories: 350 kcal per serving
- Protein: 40 g
- Carbohydrates: 8 g
- Fat: 18 g
- Fiber: 3 g

Cooking Time: 20 minutes

Serves: 4

Rating: ★★★★★

Grilled Tuna Steaks offer a luxurious dining experience, featuring the rich flavors of the sea balanced with the freshness of grilled vegetables. This dish, perfect for any special occasion, showcases the sublime texture and taste of tuna, enhanced with the simplicity of olive oil, salt, and pepper. The added zest from lemon and herbs elevates this meal to gourmet standards, making it a memorable feast.

Pan-Seared Scallops

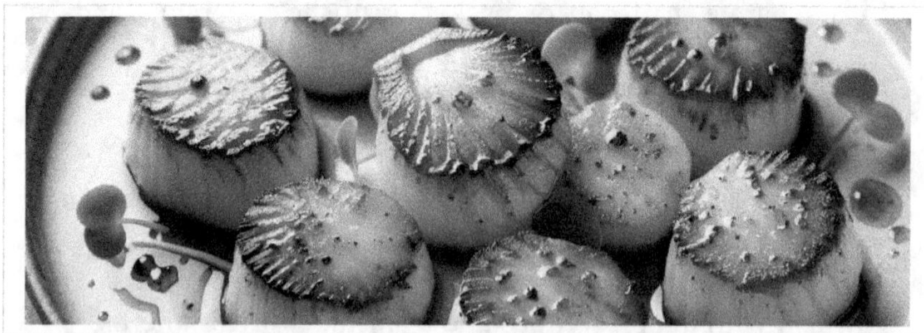

Ingredients:

- 12 large sea scallops, patted dry
- 2 tablespoons unsalted butter

- 1 tablespoon olive oil
- Salt and pepper to taste
- Optional for garnish: microgreens, lemon butter sauce

Preparation:

1. Heat a large skillet over medium-high heat. Add olive oil and butter, allowing the butter to melt.
2. Season the scallops with salt and pepper. Once the pan is hot, place the scallops in the skillet without overcrowding, ensuring they don't touch.
3. Sear the scallops for about 2 minutes on one side until they develop a golden-brown crust. Flip and cook for another 1-2 minutes on the other side until just cooked through.
4. Remove from the pan and let rest for a minute.
5. Serve on a plate, garnished with microgreens or drizzled with a lemon butter sauce.

Nutritional Values:

- Calories: 200 kcal per serving
- Protein: 20 g
- Carbohydrates: 5 g
- Fat: 10 g
- Fiber: 0 g

Cooking Time: 10 minutes

Serves: 4

Rating: ★★★★★

Pan-Seared Scallops are a testament to the beauty of simple, yet exquisite cooking. This dish, highlighting the scallops' natural sweetness with a perfect sear, is an elegant choice for any special occasion. The optional garnishes of microgreens or a lemon butter sauce add an extra layer of flavor and sophistication, making each bite a memorable experience.

Salmon Cakes

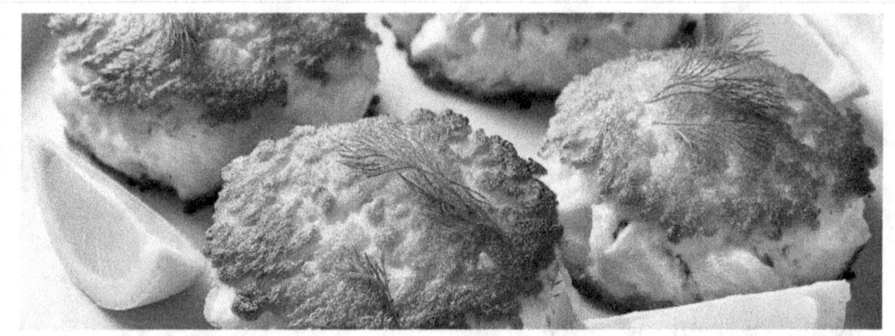

Ingredients:

- 1 lb cooked salmon, flaked
- 1 cup breadcrumbs
- 2 eggs, beaten
- 1/4 cup mayonnaise
- 2 tablespoons Dijon mustard
- 1/4 cup finely chopped green onions
- 1 tablespoon lemon juice
- Salt and pepper to taste
- Olive oil for frying
- Garnish: Lemon wedges, dill sauce or tartar sauce

Preparation:

1. In a large bowl, combine flaked salmon, breadcrumbs, eggs, mayonnaise, Dijon mustard, green onions, and lemon juice. Season with salt and pepper to taste.

2. Mix until well combined, then form into patties.

3. Heat olive oil in a skillet over medium heat. Fry the salmon cakes until golden and crispy on both sides, about 3-4 minutes per side.

4. Serve the salmon cakes hot, garnished with lemon wedges and a side of dill sauce or tartar sauce.

Nutritional Values:

- Calories: 250 kcal per serving
- Protein: 22 g
- Carbohydrates: 12 g
- Fat: 14 g
- Fiber: 1 g

Cooking Time: 20 minutes

Serves: 4

Rating: ★★★★★

Salmon Cakes are a delightful way to enjoy the rich flavors of salmon in a crispy, flavorful patty. This dish is both versatile and satisfying, making it perfect for any meal, whether it's a casual family dinner or a more sophisticated gathering. The addition of lemon wedges and a creamy sauce on the side brings a fresh and tangy element that complements the salmon perfectly.

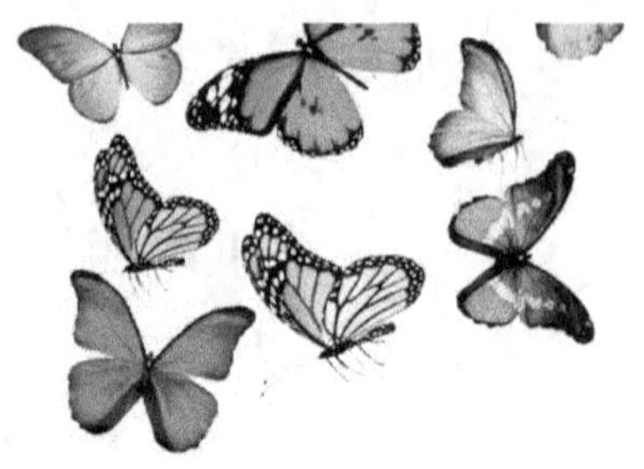

"Small changes make big differences. Each healthy choice is a victory over Hashimoto's, a step closer to reclaiming your health and vitality."

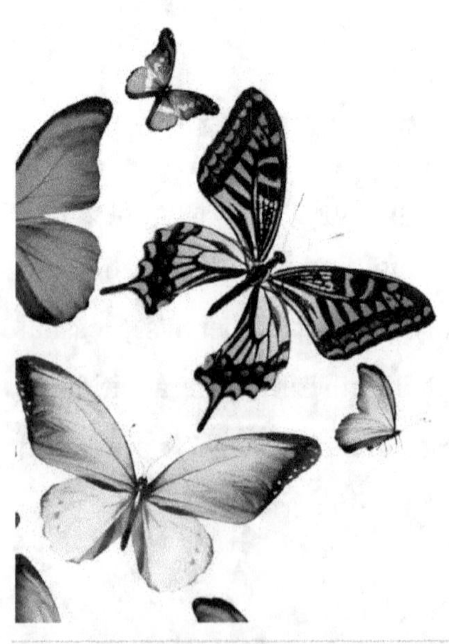

CHAPTER 9: BEEF, LAMB, AND PORK

In the Beef, Lamb, and Pork area, we explore the rich and savory world of red meats, preparing a variety of recipes that highlight the richness and diversity of these protein sources. From the strong flavors of a perfectly cooked steak to the soft succulence of slow-roasted lamb and the comforting heartiness of pig stews, each recipe is intended to highlight the meats' distinct traits and flavors. Whether you're searching for a quick weeknight supper, a slow-cooked weekend feast, or something special for a holiday, these carefully picked dishes will inspire you. Embrace culinary diversity and discover the several methods to prepare beef, lamb, and pork, with each dish offering a delightful and rewarding dining experience.

Grilled Lamb Chops

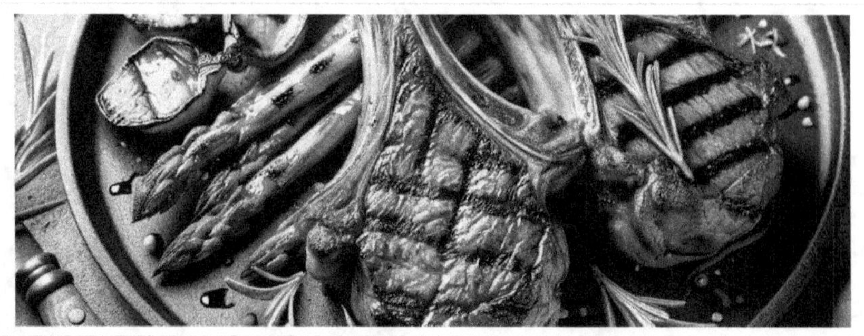

Ingredients:

- 8 lamb chops
- 2 tablespoons olive oil
- 2 cloves garlic, minced
- 1 tablespoon fresh rosemary, chopped
- Salt and pepper to taste
- Optional: Lemon wedges for serving

Preparation:

1. Preheat your grill to high heat.
2. In a small bowl, mix together olive oil, garlic, rosemary, salt, and pepper.
3. Rub the mixture over both sides of the lamb chops.
4. Place the lamb chops on the grill, cooking for about 3-4 minutes on each side for medium-rare, or until done to your liking.
5. Let the chops rest for a few minutes before serving.
6. Serve with grilled vegetables and lemon wedges if desired.

Nutritional Values:

- Calories: 310 kcal per serving
- Protein: 25 g
- Carbohydrates: 0 g
- Fat: 23 g
- Fiber: 0 g

Cooking Time: 20 minutes

Serves: 4

Rating: ★★★★★

Grilled Lamb Chops are a luxurious and flavorful meal, perfect for any special occasion. The simple marinade of olive oil, garlic, and rosemary enhances the natural flavors of the lamb, creating a dish that is both elegant and hearty. Served with a side of grilled vegetables, this meal is sure to impress.

Pork Tenderloin with Apples

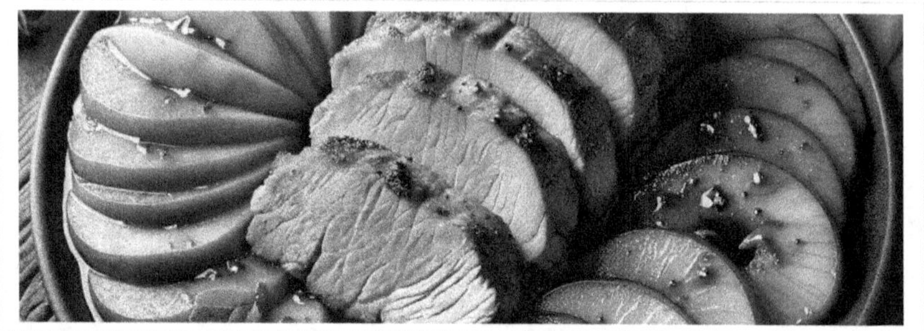

Ingredients:

- 1 pork tenderloin (about 1 lb)
- 2 tablespoons olive oil
- 3 apples, cored and sliced
- 1/4 cup apple cider vinegar
- 2 tablespoons honey
- 1 teaspoon fresh thyme, chopped
- Salt and pepper to taste

Preparation:

1. Preheat the oven to 375°F (190°C).

2. Season the pork tenderloin with salt and pepper. Heat olive oil in a large skillet over medium-high heat. Sear the tenderloin on all sides until golden brown.

3. Remove the tenderloin from the skillet and place it in a roasting pan. In the same skillet, add the sliced apples, apple cider vinegar, honey, and thyme. Cook until the apples are slightly caramelized.

4. Pour the apple mixture over the pork in the roasting pan. Bake in the preheated oven until the pork reaches an internal temperature of 145°F (63°C), about 25-30 minutes.

5. Let the pork rest for a few minutes before slicing. Serve the slices topped with the caramelized apples and drizzled with any pan juices.

Nutritional Values:

- Calories: 290 kcal per serving
- Protein: 24 g
- Carbohydrates: 22 g
- Fat: 12 g
- Fiber: 3 g

Cooking Time: 45 minutes

Serves: 4

Rating: ★★★★★

Pork Tenderloin with Apples is a delicious combination of savory and sweet flavors, making it a perfect dish for special occasions or a cozy autumn dinner. The tender pork paired with caramelized apples and a hint of thyme creates a comforting meal that's both elegant and satisfying.

Lamb Stew

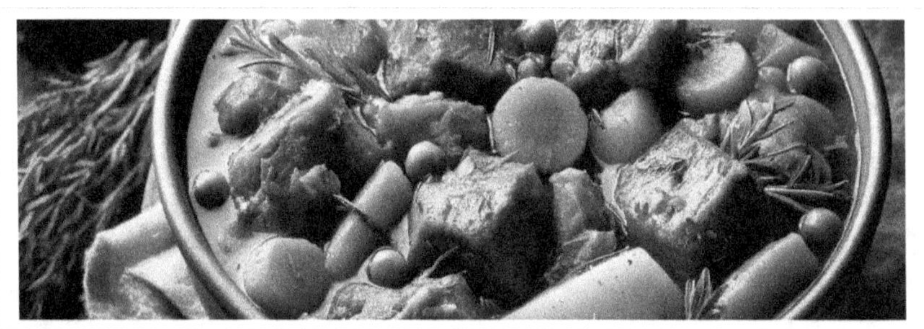

Ingredients:

- 2 lbs lamb shoulder, cut into cubes
- 3 tablespoons olive oil
- 4 carrots, peeled and sliced
- 3 potatoes, peeled and cubed
- 1 onion, chopped
- 2 cloves garlic, minced
- 4 cups beef or lamb broth
- 1 cup red wine (optional)
- 2 tablespoons tomato paste
- 1 teaspoon rosemary, chopped
- 1 teaspoon thyme, chopped
- Salt and pepper to taste
- Optional: 1 cup peas

Preparation:

1. Heat 2 tablespoons olive oil in a large pot over medium-high heat. Add lamb cubes in batches, browning on all sides. Remove lamb and set aside.
2. Reduce heat to medium. Add remaining olive oil, onion, and garlic, sautéing until softened.
3. Return lamb to the pot, adding carrots, potatoes, broth, red wine, tomato paste, rosemary, thyme, salt, and pepper. Bring to a boil, then reduce heat to low.
4. Cover and simmer for about 1.5 to 2 hours, or until lamb is tender. If using, add peas in the last 10 minutes of cooking.
5. Adjust seasoning and serve hot, garnished with additional fresh herbs if desired.

Nutritional Values:

- Calories: 450 kcal per serving
- Protein: 35 g
- Carbohydrates: 30 g
- Fat: 20 g
- Fiber: 5 g

Cooking Time: 2 hours 20 minutes

Serves: 6

Rating: ★★★★★

This Lamb Stew is a classic, comforting dish perfect for warming up on cold evenings. With tender chunks of lamb and a hearty mix of vegetables, it's a satisfying meal that's both rich in flavor and nutrients. The slow cooking process allows the flavors to meld beautifully, creating a depth of taste that makes this stew a memorable feast.

Pulled Pork Lettuce Wraps

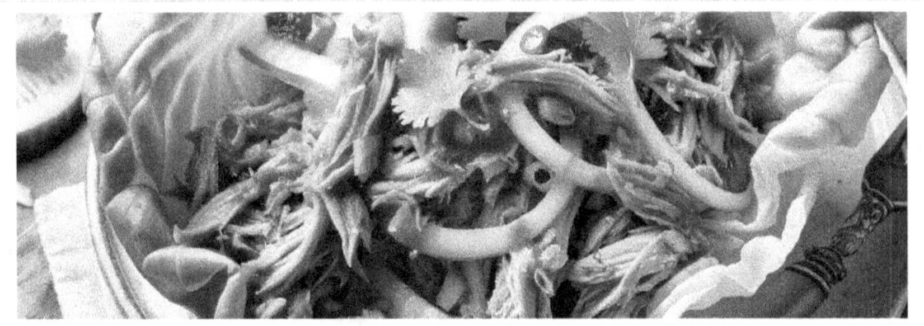

Ingredients:

- 2 lbs pork shoulder
- 1 tablespoon olive oil
- Salt and pepper to taste
- 1 cup barbecue sauce
- 1 head of iceberg or butter lettuce, leaves separated
- Optional for garnish: thinly sliced red onions, fresh cilantro, additional barbecue sauce

Preparation:

1. Season the pork shoulder with salt and pepper. In a slow cooker, add the pork and olive oil. Cover and cook on low for about 8 hours or until the pork is tender and easily shredded with a fork.

2. Remove the pork from the slow cooker and shred using two forks. Toss the shredded pork with barbecue sauce.

3. Place a spoonful of the pulled pork into the center of a lettuce leaf. If desired, top with additional barbecue sauce, sliced red onions, and fresh cilantro for extra flavor and crunch.

4. Serve immediately, allowing guests to assemble their own lettuce wraps.

Nutritional Values:

- Calories: 220 kcal per serving (2 wraps)
- Protein: 20 g
- Carbohydrates: 10 g
- Fat: 12 g
- Fiber: 1 g

Cooking Time: 8 hours 15 minutes

Serves: 6

Rating: ★★★★★

Pulled Pork Lettuce Wraps are a delightful twist on classic pulled pork, offering a lighter, healthier option without compromising on flavor.

Beef Kabobs

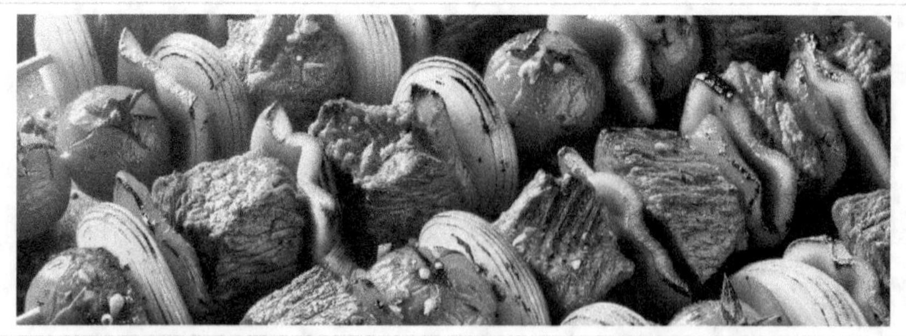

Ingredients:

- 1 lb beef sirloin, cut into 1-inch cubes
- 2 bell peppers (any color), cut into 1-inch pieces
- 1 large onion, cut into chunks
- 1 cup cherry tomatoes
- For the marinade:
    - 1/4 cup olive oil
- 1/4 cup soy sauce
- 2 tablespoons lemon juice
- 2 cloves garlic, minced
- 1 teaspoon black pepper
- 1/2 teaspoon salt

Preparation:

1. In a bowl, whisk together all marinade ingredients. Add beef cubes to the marinade, cover, and refrigerate for at least 2 hours or overnight for best flavor.
2. Preheat the grill to medium-high heat.
3. Thread the marinated beef, bell peppers, onions, and cherry tomatoes onto skewers.
4. Grill kabobs, turning occasionally, until beef reaches desired doneness and vegetables are slightly charred, about 8-10 minutes.
5. Serve hot, optionally with tzatziki sauce or garnished with fresh parsley.

Nutritional Values:

- Calories: 300 kcal per serving
- Protein: 25 g
- Carbohydrates: 10 g
- Fat: 18 g
- Fiber: 2 g

Cooking Time: 20 minutes (plus marinating time)

Serves: 4   **Rating:** ★★★★★

Beef Kabobs are a quintessential dish for grilling season, offering a delightful mix of savory beef and colorful vegetables. Marinated for depth of flavor and grilled to perfection, they make for a festive and delicious meal that's sure to please at any outdoor gathering or family dinner.

Pork Chops with Peach Salsa

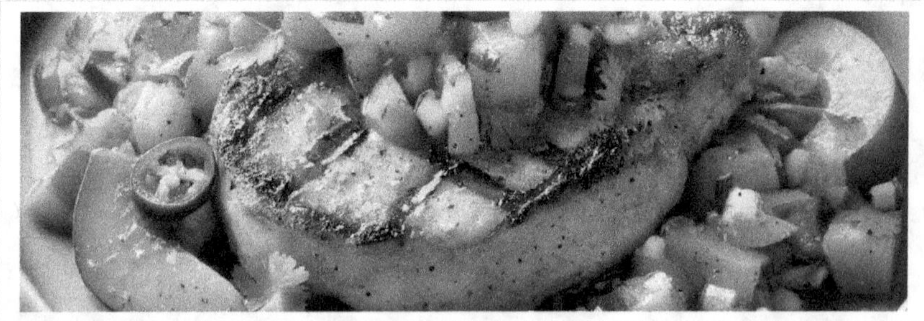

Ingredients:

- 4 pork chops
- Salt and pepper to taste
- 2 tablespoons olive oil
- **For the Peach Salsa:**
- 2 ripe peaches, diced
- 1/4 red onion, finely chopped

- 1 jalapeño, seeded and minced
- 1/4 cup cilantro, chopped
- Juice of 1 lime
- Salt to taste

Preparation:

1. Season pork chops with salt and pepper.
2. Heat olive oil in a skillet over medium-high heat. Add pork chops and cook until golden and cooked through, about 5-7 minutes per side, depending on thickness.
3. In a bowl, combine diced peaches, red onion, jalapeño, cilantro, and lime juice. Season with salt and toss gently.
4. Once pork chops are cooked, let them rest for a few minutes before serving.
5. Serve the pork chops topped with the fresh peach salsa.

Nutritional Values:

- Calories: 350 kcal per serving
- Protein: 25 g
- Carbohydrates: 15 g
- Fat: 20 g
- Fiber: 2 g

Cooking Time: 20 minutes

Serves: 4

Rating: ★★★★★

Pork Chops with Peach Salsa combine the savory taste of grilled pork with the fresh, sweet and spicy flavors of peach salsa, creating a delightful dish perfect for summer dinners. This easy-to-prepare meal brings a refreshing twist to traditional pork chops, making it a hit for any occasion.

Lamb Burgers

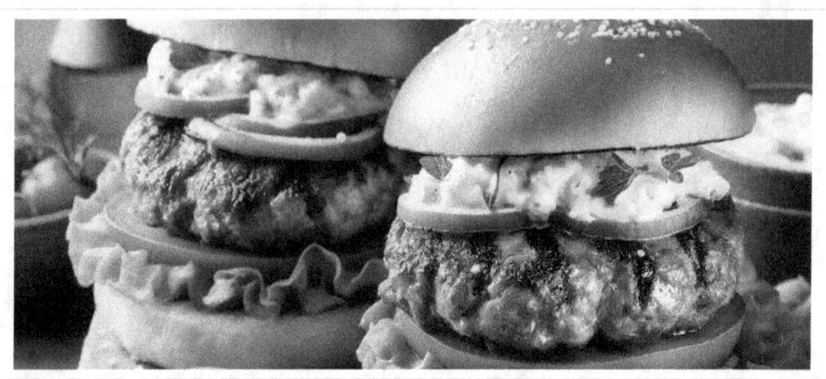

Ingredients:

- 1 lb ground lamb
- 4 burger buns, split and toasted
- 1/2 cup tzatziki sauce
- 1 tomato, sliced
- 1/2 red onion, thinly sliced
- Lettuce leaves
- Optional: crumbled feta cheese
- Salt and pepper to taste

Preparation:

1. Preheat the grill to medium-high heat.
2. Season the ground lamb with salt and pepper, then form into 4 patties.

3. Grill the patties for about 5-7 minutes on each side, or until they reach desired doneness.

4. Assemble the burgers by placing a lamb patty on the bottom half of each bun.

5. Top with lettuce, tomato slices, red onion, and a generous dollop of tzatziki sauce. Add crumbled feta cheese if using.

6. Cover with the top halves of the buns and serve immediately.

Nutritional Values:

- Calories: 550 kcal per serving
- Protein: 30 g
- Carbohydrates: 40 g
- Fat: 30 g
- Fiber: 2 g

Cooking Time: 20 minutes

Serves: 4

Rating: ★★★★★

Lamb Burgers offer a delicious twist on the traditional burger, combining the savory flavor of lamb with the cool and creamy taste of tzatziki sauce.

Steak Salad

Ingredients:

- 1 lb steak (such as ribeye, sirloin, or flank)
- 6 cups mixed greens (like arugula, spinach, and romaine)

- 1 cup cherry tomatoes, halved
- 1 cucumber, thinly sliced
- 1/2 red onion, thinly sliced
- 1 avocado, sliced
- 1/2 cup crumbled blue cheese

- Dressing:
- 3 tablespoons olive oil
- 1 tablespoon balsamic vinegar
- 1 teaspoon Dijon mustard
- Salt and pepper to taste

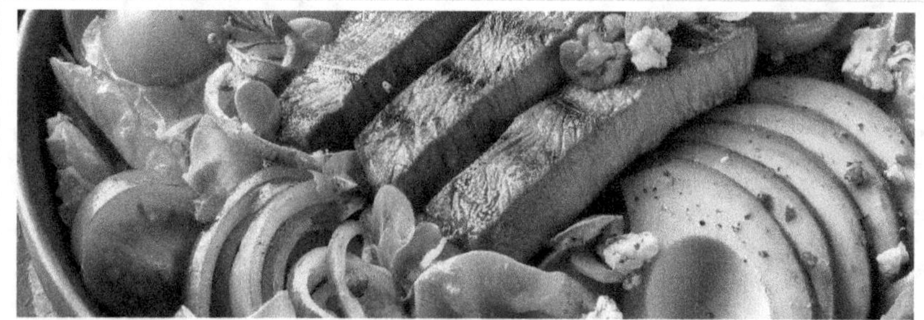

Preparation:

1. Season the steak with salt and pepper. Grill over high heat to your desired doneness, about 4-5 minutes per side for medium-rare. Let it rest for 5 minutes before slicing thinly against the grain.

2. In a large bowl, combine the mixed greens, cherry tomatoes, cucumber, and red onion.

3. Whisk together the olive oil, balsamic vinegar, Dijon mustard, salt, and pepper to make the dressing. Toss the salad with the dressing.

4. Add the sliced steak and avocado on top of the salad. Sprinkle with crumbled blue cheese.

5. Serve immediately, offering a harmonious blend of savory steak, fresh vegetables, and tangy cheese.

Nutritional Values:

- Calories: 450 kcal per serving
- Protein: 35 g
- Carbohydrates: 12 g
- Fat: 30 g
- Fiber: 6 g

Cooking Time: 20 minutes

Serves: 4

Rating: ★★★★★

This Steak Salad is a nutritious and satisfying meal that combines the hearty flavors of grilled steak with the freshness of a variety of vegetables, all complemented by the richness of blue cheese and the tanginess of balsamic dressing. It's a perfect dish for those seeking a balance of protein and greens in their diet.

Slow-Cooked Beef Ragu

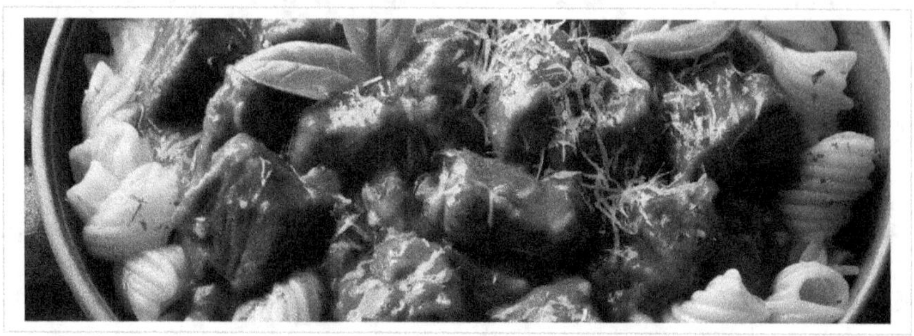

Ingredients:

- 2 lbs beef chuck roast, cut into chunks
- 1 onion, finely chopped
- 2 carrots, finely chopped
- 2 celery stalks, finely chopped
- 4 cloves garlic, minced
- 1 can (28 oz) crushed tomatoes
- 1 cup red wine
- 2 tablespoons tomato paste
- 1 teaspoon dried oregano
- 1 teaspoon dried basil
- Salt and pepper to taste
- Fresh basil or rosemary, for garnish
- Freshly grated Parmesan cheese, for serving
- Cooked pasta, for serving

Preparation:

1. Season the beef chunks with salt and pepper.
2. In a large skillet over medium-high heat, brown the beef on all sides. Transfer to a slow cooker.
3. In the same skillet, add the onion, carrots, celery, and garlic. Sauté until softened, then transfer to the slow cooker.
4. Add the crushed tomatoes, red wine, tomato paste, oregano, and basil to the slow cooker. Stir to combine.
5. Cover and cook on low for 8-10 hours or until the beef is tender and falls apart easily.
6. Serve the beef ragu over cooked pasta, garnished with fresh basil or rosemary and sprinkled with freshly grated Parmesan cheese.

Nutritional Values:

- Calories: 450 kcal per serving (including pasta)
- Protein: 35 g
- Carbohydrates: 35 g
- Fat: 20 g
- Fiber: 4 g

Cooking Time: 8-10 hours

Serves: 6

Rating: ★★★★★

This Slow-Cooked Beef Ragu is the epitome of comfort food, offering deep, rich flavors that develop through hours of slow cooking. Served over pasta and garnished with Parmesan and fresh herbs, it's a heartwarming dish perfect for a cozy night in.

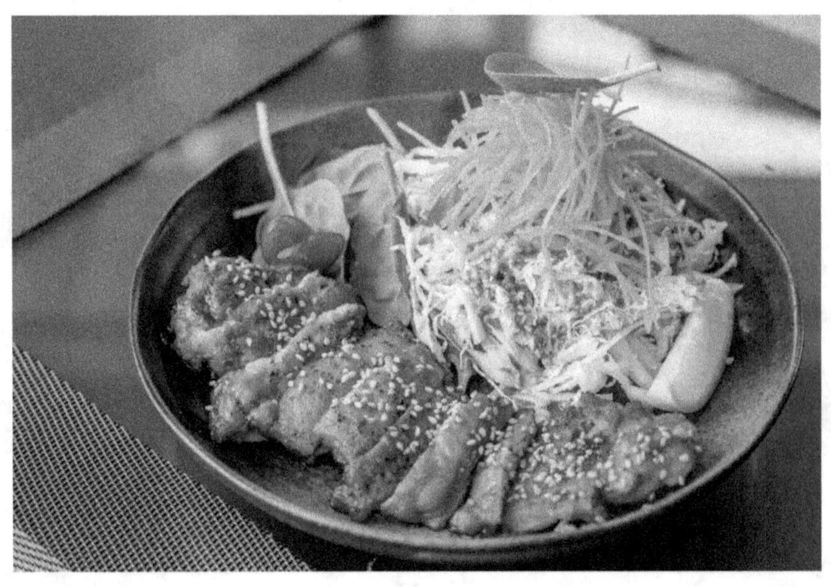

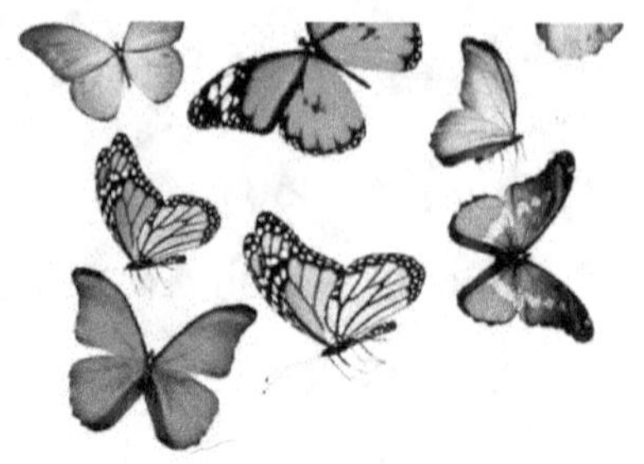

"Listen to your body; it knows what it needs to heal. Trust the journey toward health, and let your intuition guide your dietary choices."

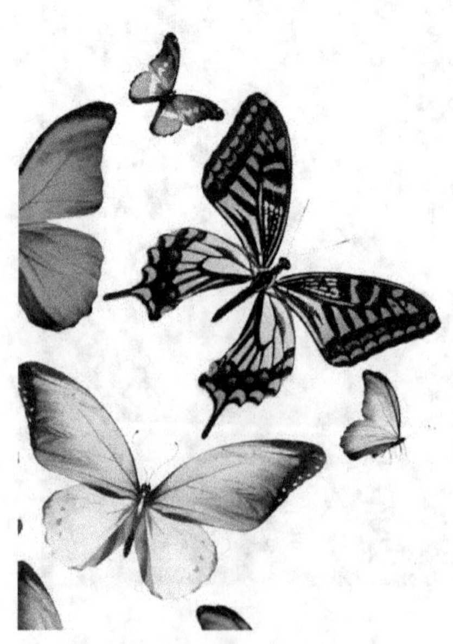

CHAPTER 10: SNACKS AND DESSERTS

Dive into the delicious world of Snacks and Desserts, where sweet and savory collide and every bite is an invitation to indulge. This section is dedicated to the pauses between meals and the sweet endings that complete each eating experience. From the crunch of precisely seasoned snack pieces to the indulgence of chocolatey desserts, each recipe is designed to satisfy your desires while also brightening your day. Whether you're looking for a quick snack to keep you going or a decadent dessert to finish your dinner, you'll find inspiration in these pages. Explore a wide selection of alternatives, from nutritious, energy-boosting snacks to decadent desserts that honor the art of pastry and baking.

Almond Butter Cups

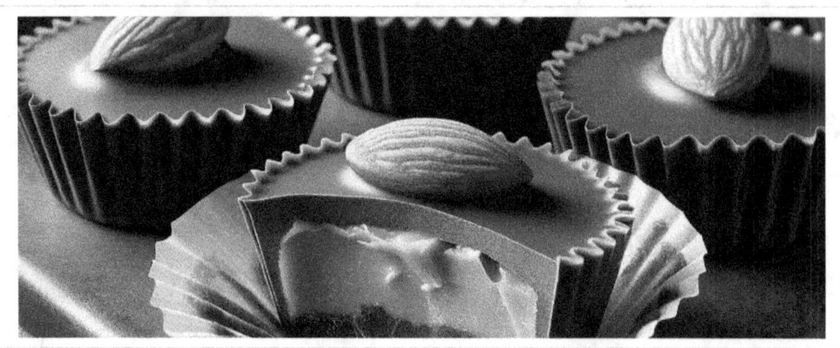

Ingredients:

- 1 cup almond butter
- 1 tablespoon coconut oil
- 2 tablespoons maple syrup (optional for sweetness)
- 1 cup dark chocolate chips
- Sea salt flakes, for garnish

Preparation:

1. Melt the dark chocolate chips and coconut oil together in a double boiler or microwave, stirring until smooth.

2. Spoon a layer of melted chocolate into the bottom of paper cupcake liners placed in a muffin tin. Freeze for about 10 minutes to set.

3. Mix the almond butter with maple syrup if desired. Spoon a small amount of almond butter over the set chocolate in each liner.

4. Cover the almond butter with another layer of melted chocolate, filling to the top of the liners.

5. Sprinkle the top with a few flakes of sea salt.

6. Freeze the almond butter cups for another 15-20 minutes or until fully set.

7. Remove from the freezer and let sit for a few minutes before serving.

Nutritional Values:

- Calories: 220 kcal per cup
- Protein: 5 g

- Carbohydrates: 12 g
- Fat: 18 g
- Fiber: 3 g

Cooking Time: 45 minutes (including setting time)

Serves: Makes 12 cups

Rating: ★★★★★

These Almond Butter Cups offer a delightful twist on the classic treat, combining the richness of almond butter with the luxurious taste of dark chocolate. A sprinkle of sea salt on top enhances the flavors, making these homemade cups a perfect balance of nutty and sweet, ideal for a satisfying snack or dessert.

Carrot Cake Energy Balls

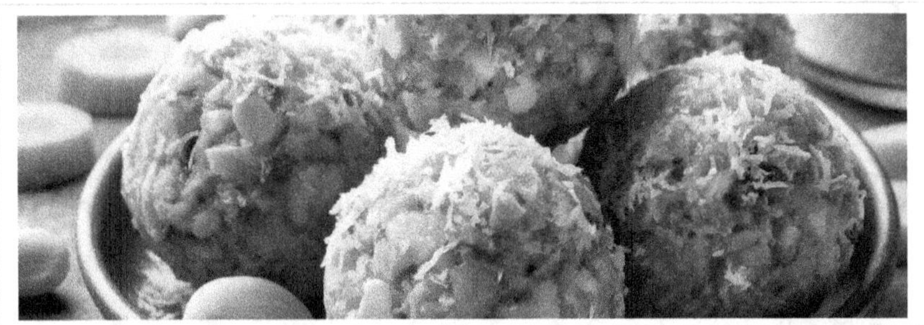

Ingredients:

- 1 cup rolled oats
- 1/2 cup grated carrot
- 1/2 cup almond butter
- 1/4 cup chopped nuts (walnuts or pecans)
- 1/4 cup raisins
- 2 tablespoons maple syrup or honey
- 1 teaspoon vanilla extract
- 1/2 teaspoon ground cinnamon

- 1/4 teaspoon ground nutmeg
- Optional for coating: shredded coconut or ground nuts

Preparation:

1. In a large bowl, combine the rolled oats, grated carrot, almond butter, chopped nuts, raisins, maple syrup or honey, vanilla extract, cinnamon, and nutmeg. Mix until well combined.
2. Refrigerate the mixture for about 30 minutes to firm up, making it easier to handle.
3. Roll the mixture into bite-sized balls, about 1 inch in diameter.
4. If desired, roll each ball in shredded coconut or ground nuts for an extra layer of flavor and texture.
5. Store the energy balls in an airtight container in the refrigerator.

Nutritional Values:

- Calories: 100 kcal per ball
- Protein: 3 g
- Carbohydrates: 12 g
- Fat: 5 g
- Fiber: 2 g

Cooking Time: 45 minutes (including chilling time)

Serves: Makes 12-15 balls   **Rating:** ★★★★★

These Carrot Cake Energy Balls are a delicious and healthy snack, packed with the flavors of carrot cake and the nutritional benefits of oats, nuts, and carrots. Perfect for on-the-go snacking or as a post-workout energy boost, they offer a wholesome alternative to traditional sweets.

Coconut Flour Cookies

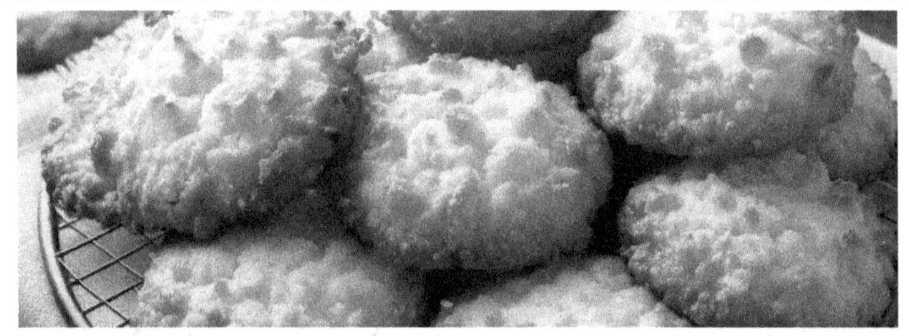

Ingredients:

- 1/2 cup coconut flour
- 1/4 cup melted coconut oil
- 1/4 cup maple syrup or honey
- 2 eggs
- 1/2 teaspoon vanilla extract
- 1/4 teaspoon salt
- Optional: Chocolate chips or nuts for mix-ins

Preparation:

1. Preheat the oven to 350°F (175°C) and line a baking sheet with parchment paper.
2. In a mixing bowl, combine coconut flour, melted coconut oil, maple syrup or honey, eggs, vanilla extract, and salt. Stir until well combined. If using, fold in chocolate chips or nuts.

3. Drop tablespoon-sized scoops of dough onto the prepared baking sheet. Flatten each scoop slightly with the back of the spoon, as the cookies will not spread much during baking.

4. Bake for 12-15 minutes, or until the edges start to turn golden brown.

5. Remove from the oven and let cool on the baking sheet for a few minutes before transferring to a wire rack to cool completely.

Nutritional Values:

- Calories: 90 kcal per cookie
- Protein: 2 g
- Carbohydrates: 8 g
- Fat: 6 g
- Fiber: 2 g

Cooking Time: 30 minutes

Serves: Makes 12 cookies

Rating: ★★★★★

These Coconut Flour Cookies are a delightful, gluten-free treat that combines the natural sweetness of coconut with the richness of coconut oil for a tender, flavorful snack.

Baked Apple Chips

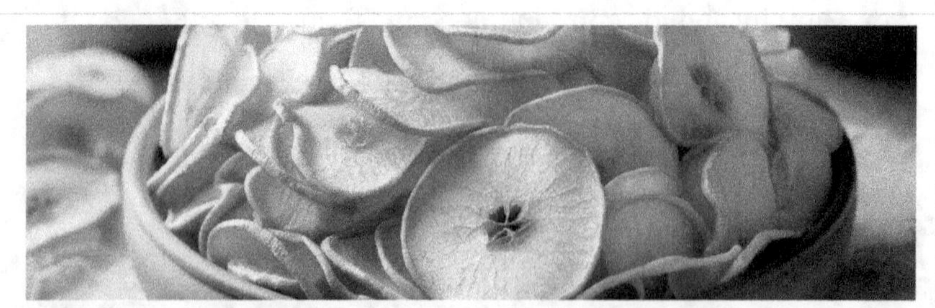

Ingredients:

- 2 large apples (such as Fuji or Granny Smith)
- Cinnamon (optional)

Preparation:

1. Preheat your oven to 200°F (93°C). Line two baking sheets with parchment paper.
2. Core the apples and slice them very thinly using a mandoline slicer or a sharp knife.
3. Arrange the apple slices in a single layer on the prepared baking sheets. If desired, sprinkle with cinnamon for added flavor.
4. Bake for 1-2 hours, flipping the slices halfway through, until the apple slices are dried out and crispy.
5. Let the apple chips cool completely on the baking sheets to crisp up further.

Nutritional Values:

- Calories: 50 kcal per serving (about 1 apple's worth of chips)
- Protein: 0 g
- Carbohydrates: 13 g
- Fat: 0 g
- Fiber: 2 g

Cooking Time: 2 hours

Serves: Makes 4 servings

Rating: ★★★★★

Baked Apple Chips are a simple, healthy snack that captures the essence of apples in a light, crunchy form. With no added sugars and the optional hint of cinnamon, they're an ideal choice for those looking for a naturally sweet treat that's both delicious and nutritious.

Avocado Chocolate Mousse

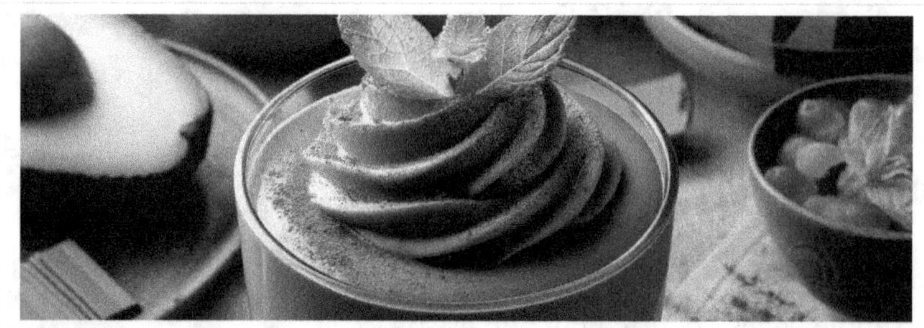

Ingredients:

- 2 ripe avocados, peeled and pitted
- 1/4 cup cocoa powder
- 1/4 cup maple syrup or honey
- 1/2 teaspoon vanilla extract
- A pinch of salt
- Optional garnishes: mint leaves, dark chocolate shavings, fresh berries

Preparation:

1. In a blender or food processor, combine the avocados, cocoa powder, maple syrup (or honey), vanilla extract, and a pinch of salt. Blend until the mixture is smooth and creamy.

2. Taste and adjust sweetness if necessary. If the mousse is too thick, you can add a tablespoon of almond milk or water to reach the desired consistency.

3. Divide the mousse into serving glasses or bowls and refrigerate for at least 1 hour to set.

4. Before serving, garnish with mint leaves, dark chocolate shavings, or fresh berries for an added touch of elegance and flavor.

Nutritional Values:

- Calories: 220 kcal per serving
- Protein: 3 g
- Carbohydrates: 25 g
- Fat: 14 g
- Fiber: 7 g

Cooking Time: 15 minutes + chilling time

Serves: 4   **Rating:** ★★★★★

This Avocado Chocolate Mousse is a decadent yet healthy dessert, utilizing the creaminess of avocados to create a luxurious texture without dairy. The rich chocolate flavor, enhanced with natural sweeteners and a hint of vanilla, makes for a sophisticated treat that's perfect for impressing guests or enjoying a guilt-free indulgence.

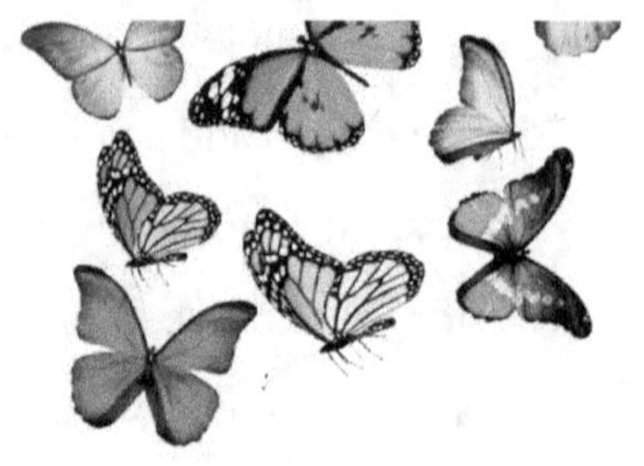

"You are what you eat, so choose wisely and fuel your body to fight Hashimoto's with all the nutrients it needs to recover and thrive."

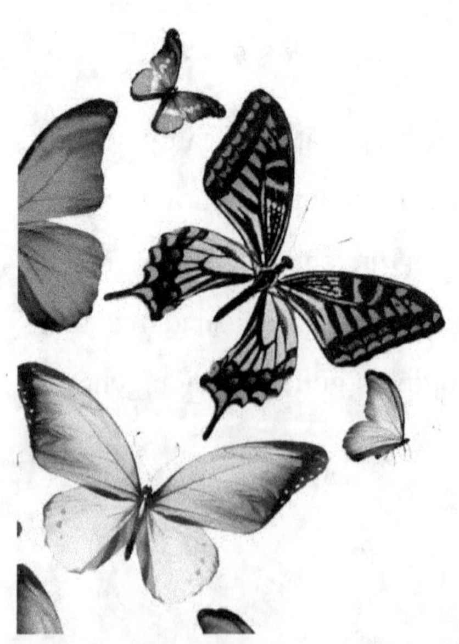

CHAPTER 11: PIZZA

Take a gastronomic journey through the world of pizza, a renowned dish that spans borders and combines a symphony of flavors on a wonderful dough. This area showcases pizza's flexibility, from the classic Margherita, which pays homage to traditional Italian traditions, to creative variants that test the boundaries of flavor and texture. Discover recipes for various tastes, including thin-crust lovers, deep-dish fans, and those looking for gluten-free or plant-based options. Each recipe is intended to encourage both rookie and experienced cooks to experiment with different toppings, sauces, and cheeses when preparing pizza. Whether you want to reproduce the ambiance of a Naples pizzeria or simply bring the joy of homemade pizza into your kitchen, this collection will help you master the technique and share your love of pizza with friends and family. Let us raise a slice to pizza's limitless possibilities, inviting everyone to enjoy its delectable combinations of flavors and textures.

Cauliflower Crust Margherita Pizza

Ingredients:

- 1 head of cauliflower, riced and cooked
- 1 egg, beaten
- 1/2 cup grated Parmesan cheese
- Salt and pepper to taste
- 1/2 cup tomato sauce
- 1 tomato, sliced
- 1 cup fresh mozzarella cheese, sliced
- Fresh basil leaves, for garnish

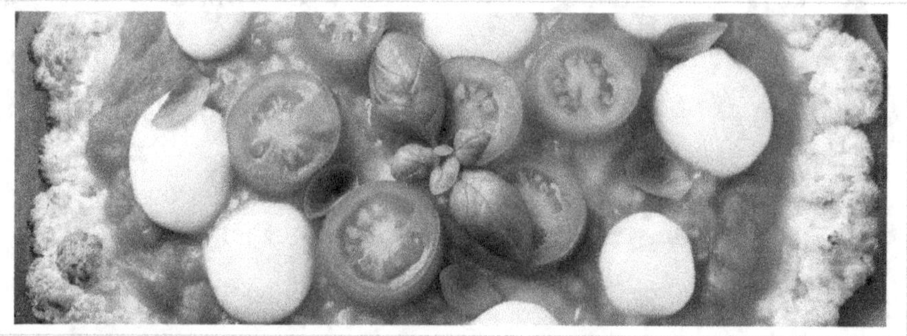

Preparation:

1. Preheat your oven to 400°F (200°C). Line a baking sheet with parchment paper.

2. Mix the cooked cauliflower rice with the egg, Parmesan, salt, and pepper. Press the mixture onto the lined baking sheet, forming a pizza base.

3. Bake the crust for 20 minutes, or until it's golden and firm.

4. Spread tomato sauce over the baked crust, then top with tomato and mozzarella slices.

5. Return to the oven and bake for another 10 minutes, until the cheese is bubbly and slightly golden.

6. Garnish with fresh basil leaves before serving.

Nutritional Values:

- Calories: 250 kcal per serving
- Protein: 15 g
- Carbohydrates: 15 g
- Fat: 15 g
- Fiber: 4 g

Cooking Time: 40 minutes

Serves: 2

Rating: ★★★★★

This Cauliflower Crust Margherita Pizza offers a delicious and healthy twist on the traditional pizza, featuring a crispy cauliflower crust topped with classic Margherita ingredients. It's a flavorful, gluten-free option that doesn't compromise on taste or texture.

Spinach and Goat Cheese Pizza

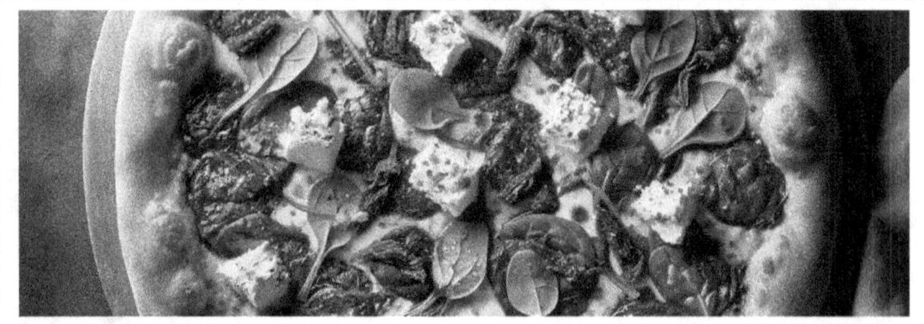

Ingredients:

- Pizza dough (store-bought or homemade)
- 1 tablespoon olive oil, plus more for drizzling
- 2 cups fresh spinach leaves
- 1 cup crumbled goat cheese

- 1/2 cup caramelized onions
- 1/4 cup sun-dried tomatoes, chopped
- Crushed red pepper flakes (optional)
- Salt and pepper to taste

Preparation:

1. Preheat your oven as directed by the pizza dough instructions, typically around 475°F (245°C).

2. Roll out the pizza dough on a baking sheet lined with parchment paper. Brush the surface with olive oil.

3. Evenly spread the spinach leaves over the dough, followed by caramelized onions and sun-dried tomatoes.

4. Scatter crumbled goat cheese across the pizza. Season with salt, pepper, and crushed red pepper flakes if desired.

5. Bake in the preheated oven until the crust is golden and crispy, about 12-15 minutes.

6. Once out of the oven, drizzle with a little more olive oil before serving.

Nutritional Values:

- Calories: 300 kcal per slice (estimation varies based on dough type and toppings quantity)
- Protein: 12 g
- Carbohydrates: 35 g
- Fat: 14 g
- Fiber: 2 g

Cooking Time: 30 minutes (including preparation and baking time)

Serves: 4   **Rating:** ★★★★★

This Spinach and Goat Cheese Pizza is a delightful blend of creamy goat cheese and fresh spinach on a crispy crust, enhanced by the sweetness of caramelized onions and the tang of sun-dried tomatoes. It's a gourmet twist on traditional pizza, perfect for those seeking a sophisticated yet comforting meal.

Chicken Pesto Pizza

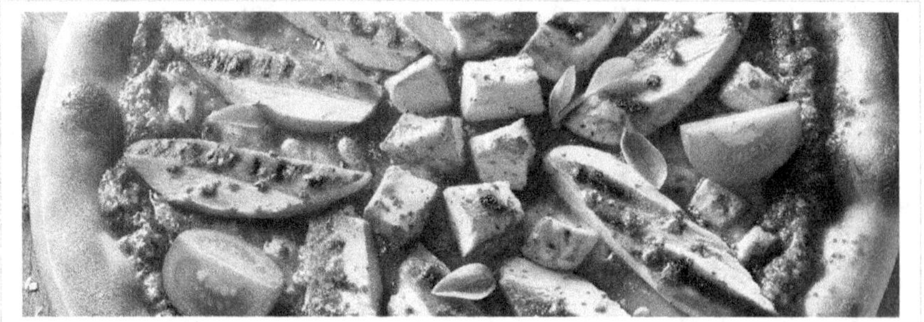

Ingredients:

- 1 pizza dough (store-bought or homemade)
- 1/2 cup pesto sauce
- 1 cup cooked chicken, sliced or shredded
- 1 cup mozzarella cheese, shredded
- 1/2 cup cherry tomatoes, halved
- 1/4 cup Parmesan cheese, grated
- Red pepper flakes (optional)
- Fresh basil leaves, for garnish

Preparation:

1. Preheat your oven to the temperature specified by your pizza dough instructions, typically around 475°F (245°C).
2. Roll out the pizza dough on a baking sheet lined with parchment paper.
3. Spread the pesto sauce evenly over the dough, leaving a small border around the edges.
4. Top with cooked chicken, mozzarella cheese, and cherry tomatoes.
5. Sprinkle with Parmesan cheese and red pepper flakes if using.
6. Bake in the preheated oven until the crust is golden and the cheese is bubbly, about 12-15 minutes.
7. Garnish with fresh basil leaves before serving.

Nutritional Values:

- Calories: 320 kcal per slice (estimation varies based on dough type and toppings quantity)
- Protein: 18 g
- Carbohydrates: 25 g
- Fat: 16 g
- Fiber: 1 g

Cooking Time: 30 minutes (including preparation and baking time)

Serves: 4   **Rating:** ★★★★★

Chicken Pesto Pizza combines the rich, herby flavor of pesto with the savory goodness of chicken and the freshness of tomatoes, all melted together with mozzarella and Parmesan cheese on a crispy crust. This pizza is a flavorful twist on traditional toppings, perfect for a quick dinner or a special weekend treat.

Mushroom and Arugula Pizza

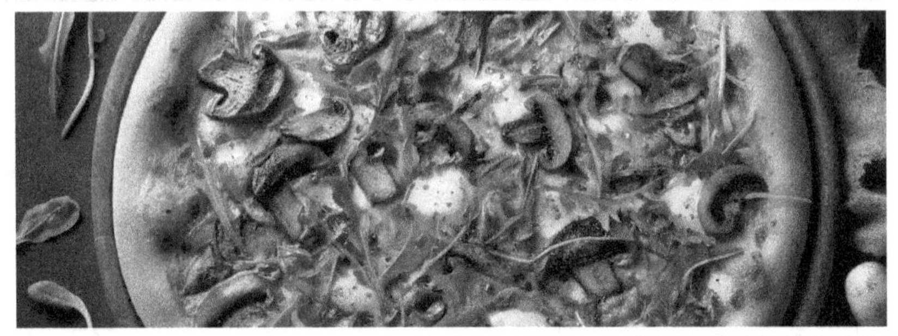

Ingredients:

- 1 pizza dough (store-bought or homemade)
- 1/2 cup pizza sauce
- 1 cup mozzarella cheese, shredded
- 1 cup mushrooms, sliced and sautéed
- 1 cup arugula, fresh
- 1/4 cup goat cheese or Parmesan cheese, crumbled
- Drizzle of truffle oil or balsamic reduction (optional)

Preparation:

1. Preheat your oven according to the pizza dough instructions, typically around 475°F (245°C).
2. Roll out the pizza dough on a baking sheet lined with parchment paper.

3. Spread the pizza sauce evenly over the dough, leaving a small border around the edges.

4. Top with shredded mozzarella cheese and sautéed mushrooms.

5. Bake in the preheated oven until the crust is golden and the cheese is bubbly, about 12-15 minutes.

6. Remove from the oven and immediately top with fresh arugula and crumbled goat cheese or Parmesan.

7. Drizzle with truffle oil or balsamic reduction if desired before serving.

Nutritional Values:

- Calories: 320 kcal per slice (estimation varies based on dough type and toppings quantity)
- Protein: 15 g
- Carbohydrates: 35 g
- Fat: 15 g
- Fiber: 2 g

Cooking Time: 30 minutes (including preparation and baking time)

Serves: 4

Rating: ★★★★★

This Mushroom and Arugula Pizza combines the earthy flavors of sautéed mushrooms with the peppery freshness of arugula, all on a crispy crust. The addition of creamy mozzarella and tangy goat cheese or Parmesan adds depth, while a drizzle of truffle oil or balsamic reduction can bring an extra layer of gourmet flair to this delightful meal.

BBQ Chicken Pizza

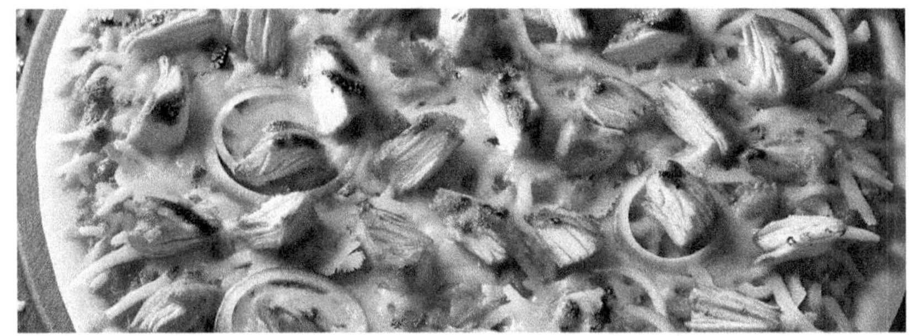

Ingredients:

- 1 pizza dough (store-bought or homemade)
- 1/2 cup BBQ sauce
- 1 cup cooked chicken, shredded
- 1/2 red onion, thinly sliced
- 1 cup mozzarella cheese, shredded
- 1/2 cup cheddar cheese, shredded
- Fresh cilantro leaves, for garnish

Preparation:

1. Preheat your oven according to the pizza dough instructions, typically around 475°F (245°C).
2. Roll out the pizza dough on a baking sheet lined with parchment paper.
3. Spread the BBQ sauce evenly over the dough, leaving a small border around the edges.
4. Top with shredded chicken, sliced red onion, mozzarella cheese, and cheddar cheese.

5. Bake in the preheated oven until the crust is golden and the cheese is bubbly, about 12-15 minutes.

6. Garnish with fresh cilantro leaves before serving.

Nutritional Values:

- Calories: 350 kcal per slice (estimation varies based on dough type and toppings quantity)
- Protein: 20 g
- Carbohydrates: 35 g
- Fat: 15 g
- Fiber: 2 g

Cooking Time: 30 minutes (including preparation and baking time)

Serves: 4   **Rating:** ★★★★★

BBQ Chicken Pizza is a delightful fusion of tangy BBQ sauce, savory chicken, and melted cheese, all on a crispy crust. It's a perfect meal for anyone craving the comfort of pizza with the bold flavors of barbecue. The addition of fresh cilantro adds a refreshing touch to this popular dish.

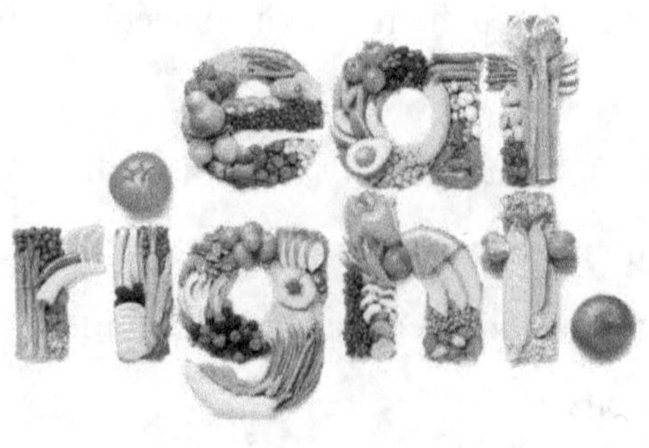

CHAPTER 12: CASSEROLE

Casseroles are the archetypal comfort dish, ideal for family meals, potlucks, and any event requiring a hearty meal. This section delves into a range of casserole recipes, ranging from traditional favorites like lasagna and shepherd's pie to creative meals that will introduce new flavors and textures to your table. Each recipe is intended to be simple and convenient, with many allowing for preparation, making it suitable for busy weeknights or casual weekend gatherings. Whether you prefer something cheesy, veggie-packed, meaty, or even sweet, there is a casserole for everyone. Dive in and see how these one-dish miracles can simplify and satisfy your eating experience, with layers of ingredients baked together to produce a symphony of tastes that are both nourishing and delicious.

Chicken Broccoli Casserole

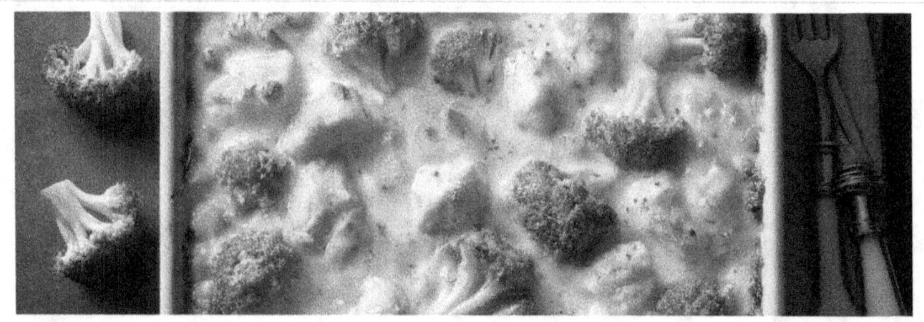

Ingredients:

- 2 cups cooked chicken, shredded
- 3 cups broccoli florets, lightly steamed
- 1 can (10.5 oz) cream of chicken soup
- 1 cup sour cream
- 1 cup cheddar cheese, shredded
- 1/2 cup milk
- 1 teaspoon garlic powder
- Salt and pepper to taste
- 1/2 cup breadcrumbs (optional for topping)
- 1 tablespoon melted butter (optional for breadcrumb topping)

Preparation:

1. Preheat your oven to 350°F (175°C).
2. In a large mixing bowl, combine the cream of chicken soup, sour cream, cheddar cheese, milk, garlic powder, salt, and pepper. Stir until well mixed.
3. Fold in the cooked chicken and steamed broccoli until they are coated with the sauce mixture.
4. Transfer the mixture to a greased baking dish.
5. If using, mix breadcrumbs with melted butter and sprinkle over the top of the casserole.
6. Bake for 25-30 minutes, or until the casserole is bubbly and the top is golden brown.
7. Let it cool for a few minutes before serving.

Nutritional Values:

- Calories: 350 kcal per serving
- Protein: 25 g
- Carbohydrates: 15 g
- Fat: 20 g
- Fiber: 2 g

Cooking Time: 55 minutes (including prep time)

Serves: 6

Rating: ★★★★★

This Chicken Broccoli Casserole is a comforting and hearty dish that combines the savory flavors of chicken and broccoli in a creamy, cheesy sauce. Topped with a golden breadcrumb crust, it's a perfect meal for a cozy night in or a family dinner.

Eggplant Parmesan Casserole

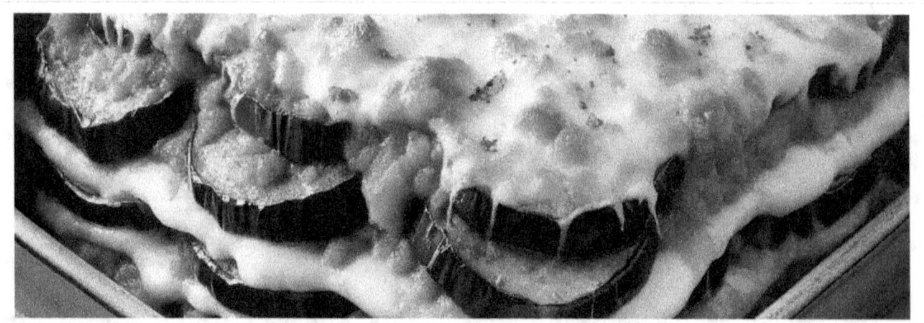

Ingredients:

- 2 large eggplants, sliced into 1/4-inch rounds
- Salt, for drawing out water from eggplant
- 2 cups breadcrumbs
- 1 cup grated Parmesan cheese, divided
- 2 eggs, beaten

- 2 cups marinara sauce
- 2 cups shredded mozzarella cheese
- Olive oil, for brushing
- Fresh basil, for garnish

Preparation:

1. Preheat your oven to 375°F (190°C). Sprinkle salt over the eggplant slices and let them sit for about 20 minutes to draw out moisture. Rinse and pat dry.
2. Combine breadcrumbs and half of the Parmesan cheese in a shallow dish. Dip each eggplant slice in the beaten eggs, then coat with the breadcrumb mixture.
3. Place the breaded eggplant slices on a baking sheet lined with parchment paper. Lightly brush each slice with olive oil. Bake for 25 minutes, flipping halfway through, until golden and crispy.
4. In a casserole dish, spread a thin layer of marinara sauce. Layer half of the baked eggplant slices over the sauce. Cover with more sauce, then sprinkle with half of the mozzarella cheese. Repeat the layers with the remaining ingredients.
5. Top with the remaining Parmesan cheese. Bake for 20-25 minutes, or until the cheese is bubbly and golden.
6. Let cool for a few minutes before garnishing with fresh basil and serving.

Nutritional Values:

- Calories: 380 kcal per serving
- Protein: 20 g
- Carbohydrates: 35 g
- Fat: 20 g
- Fiber: 6 g

Cooking Time: 1 hour 15 minutes

Serves: 6

Rating: ★★★★★

Eggplant Parmesan Casserole is a hearty, comforting dish that brings together the classic flavors of Italy in a vegetarian-friendly way. With layers of crispy baked eggplant, tangy marinara sauce, and gooey cheese, it's a satisfying meal that's perfect for a cozy dinner at home.

Zucchini Lasagna

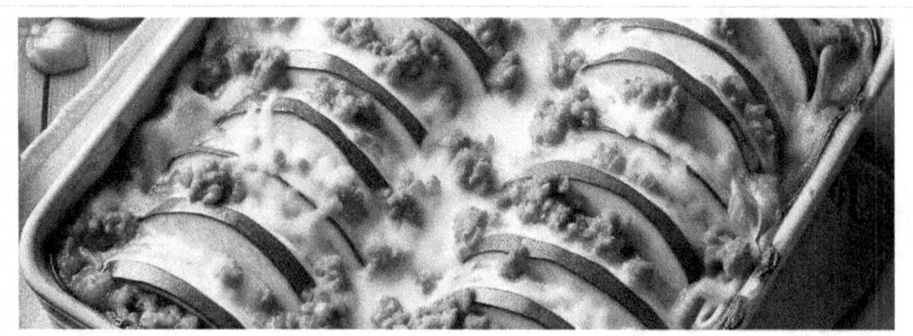

Ingredients:

- 4 large zucchinis, sliced lengthwise into thin strips
- 1 lb ground beef or a vegetarian substitute
- 1 jar (24 oz) marinara sauce
- 15 oz ricotta cheese

- 1 egg

- 2 cups shredded mozzarella cheese

- 1/2 cup grated Parmesan cheese

- 2 tablespoons fresh basil, chopped

- Salt and pepper to taste

Preparation:

1. Preheat your oven to 375°F (190°C). Salt the zucchini slices and set aside for 10 minutes to draw out moisture. Pat dry with paper towels.

2. In a skillet over medium heat, cook the ground beef until browned. Drain excess fat and stir in marinara sauce. Simmer for 10 minutes.

3. In a bowl, mix ricotta cheese, egg, and basil. Season with salt and pepper.

4. In a baking dish, layer zucchini slices, ricotta mixture, meat sauce, and mozzarella cheese. Repeat layers and top with Parmesan cheese.

5. Cover with foil and bake for 30 minutes. Remove foil and bake for an additional 20 minutes until cheese is golden and bubbly.

6. Let the lasagna rest for 10 minutes before serving.

Nutritional Values:

- Calories: 320 kcal per serving
- Protein: 25 g
- Carbohydrates: 12 g
- Fat: 20 g
- Fiber: 2 g

Cooking Time: 1 hour 10 minutes

Serves: 8   **Rating:** ★★★★★

Zucchini Lasagna is a nutritious and flavorful alternative to traditional lasagna, perfect for those seeking a low-carb, gluten-free meal without compromising on taste. This dish layers zucchini with rich sauces and cheeses, offering a delicious way to enjoy a classic comfort food.

Sweet Potato Casserole

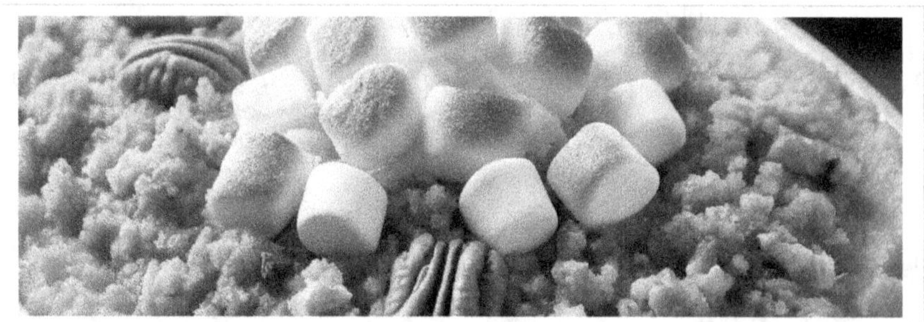

Ingredients:

- 4 cups mashed sweet potatoes
- 1/2 cup sugar
- 2 eggs, beaten
- 1/2 cup milk
- 1/4 cup butter, melted
- 1 teaspoon vanilla extract
- **For the topping:**

- 1/2 cup brown sugar
- 1/3 cup flour
- 3 tablespoons butter, softened
- 1/2 cup chopped pecans or walnuts
- 1 cup mini marshmallows (optional)

Preparation:

1. Preheat your oven to 350°F (175°C).
2. In a large bowl, mix together the mashed sweet potatoes, sugar, eggs, milk, melted butter, and vanilla extract until well combined.
3. Pour the sweet potato mixture into a greased baking dish.
4. In a separate bowl, mix the brown sugar, flour, softened butter, and chopped nuts to make the crumble topping. Sprinkle evenly over the sweet potato mixture.
5. Bake for 25 minutes. If using marshmallows, add them on top of the casserole during the last 10 minutes of baking, until golden and puffed.
6. Serve warm as a delightful side dish.

Nutritional Values:

- Calories: 300 kcal per serving
- Protein: 4 g
- Carbohydrates: 50 g
- Fat: 10 g
- Fiber: 3 g

Cooking Time: 35 minutes

Serves: 8   **Rating:** ★★★★★

Sweet Potato Casserole is a classic dish that blends the natural sweetness of sweet potatoes with a crunchy, nutty topping, and optional marshmallows for an extra layer of indulgence. It's a festive, comforting side perfect for special occasions, offering a delicious combination of flavors and textures.

Tuna Noodle Casserole

Ingredients:

- 8 ounces egg noodles, cooked and drained
- 2 cans (5 ounces each) tuna in water, drained and flaked
- 1 cup frozen peas, thawed
- 1 can (10.5 ounces) cream of mushroom soup
- 1/2 cup milk
- 1/2 cup sour cream
- 1 cup cheddar cheese, shredded
- 1/2 cup breadcrumbs or cracker crumbs
- 2 tablespoons butter, melted
- Salt and pepper to taste

Preparation:

1. Preheat your oven to 375°F (190°C). Grease a 9x13 inch baking dish.

2. In a large bowl, combine the cooked egg noodles, flaked tuna, and thawed peas.

3. In another bowl, whisk together the cream of mushroom soup, milk, and sour cream. Season with salt and pepper.

4. Pour the soup mixture over the noodle mixture and stir until well combined. Stir in half of the shredded cheddar cheese.

5. Transfer the mixture to the prepared baking dish. Top with the remaining cheddar cheese.

6. In a small bowl, mix the breadcrumbs or cracker crumbs with melted butter. Sprinkle this mixture over the casserole.

7. Bake for 25-30 minutes, or until the topping is golden brown and the casserole is bubbly.

8. Let it cool for a few minutes before serving.

Nutritional Values:

- Calories: 350 kcal per serving
- Protein: 20 g
- Carbohydrates: 35 g
- Fat: 15 g
- Fiber: 2 g

Cooking Time: 45 minutes

Serves: 6

Rating: ★★★★★

Tuna Noodle Casserole is a beloved comfort food classic that combines simple ingredients into a warm, hearty dish. With its creamy sauce, tender noodles, and savory tuna, topped with a crispy breadcrumb layer, it's a satisfying meal that brings back memories of home-cooked dinners.

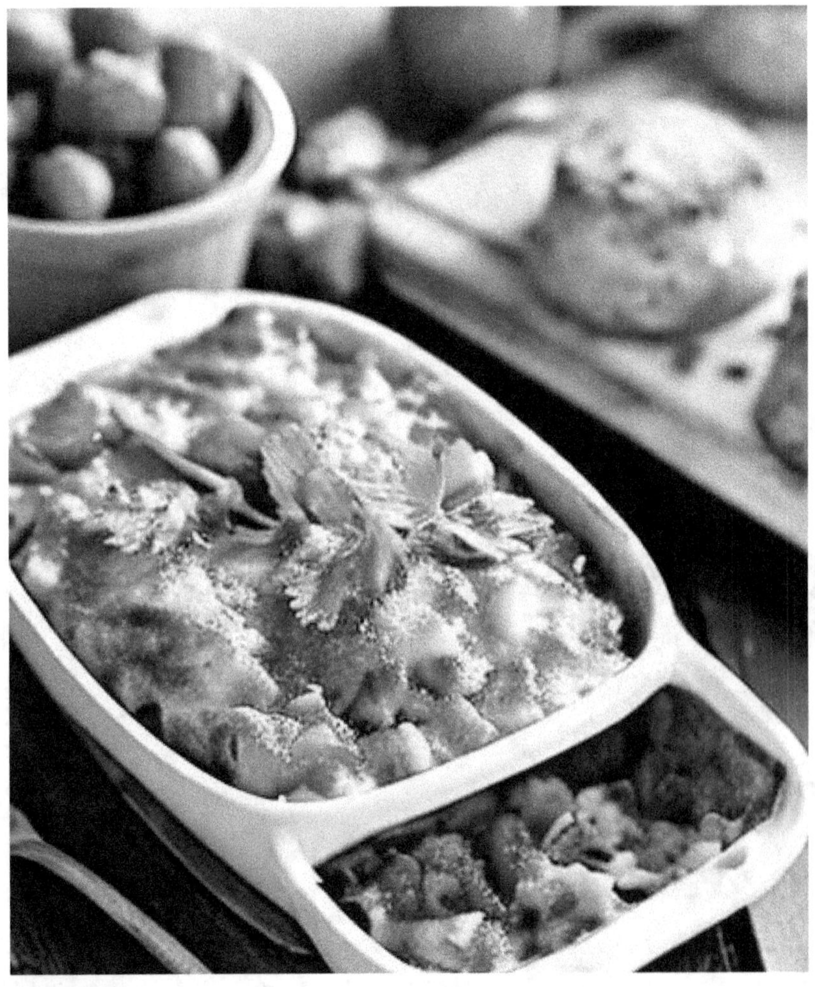

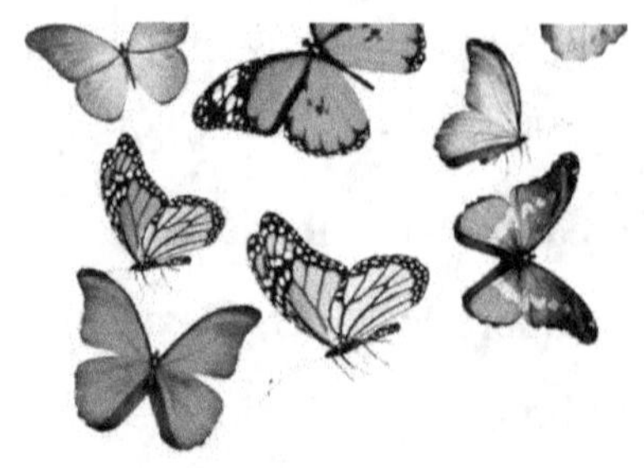

"Your health is an investment, not an expense. Investing in nutritious foods will pay off with interest in the form of better health and a brighter future."

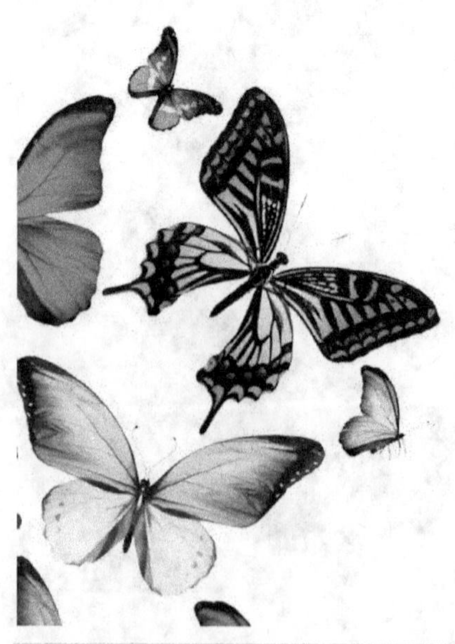

CHAPTER 13: PIE

Dive into the versatile world of pies, where sweet meets savory across a range of delicious recipes. From classic fruit pies bursting with seasonal flavors to hearty savory pies perfect for any meal, this section offers a pie for every occasion. Discover the joys of baking with easy-to-follow recipes that promise to delight your taste buds and impress your guests. Whether you're a seasoned baker or new to the art, find your next favorite pie here.

Shepherd's Pie

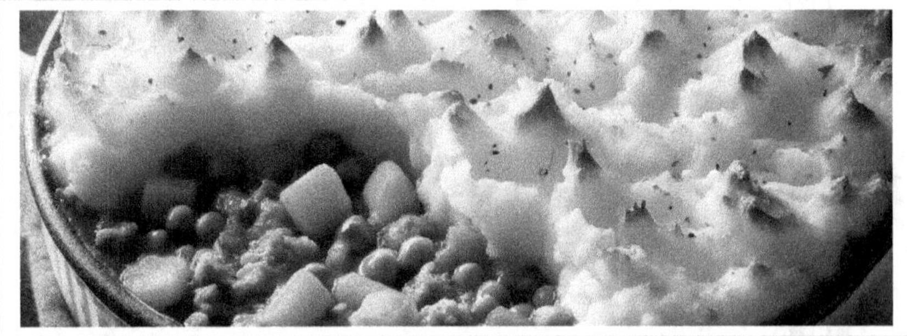

Ingredients:

- 1 lb ground lamb (or beef for Cottage Pie)
- 1 onion, chopped
- 2 carrots, diced
- 1 cup frozen peas
- 2 cloves garlic, minced

- 1 cup beef broth
- 2 tablespoons tomato paste
- 1 tablespoon Worcestershire sauce
- Salt and pepper to taste
- 2 lbs potatoes, peeled and cubed
- 1/4 cup milk
- 2 tablespoons butter
- 1/2 cup grated cheddar cheese (optional)

Preparation:

1. Boil potatoes in salted water until tender. Mash with milk and butter. Season with salt and pepper. Set aside.
2. Brown the meat in a skillet. Add onions, carrots, and garlic. Cook until softened.
3. Stir in tomato paste, Worcestershire sauce, and beef broth. Bring to a simmer, then add peas. Cook until thickened.
4. Transfer the meat mixture to a baking dish. Top with mashed potatoes. Sprinkle with cheese if using.
5. Bake at 400°F (200°C) for about 20 minutes, or until the top is golden.
6. Let it rest before serving.

Nutritional Values:

- Calories: 350 kcal per serving
- Protein: 22 g
- Carbohydrates: 35 g
- Fat: 15 g
- Fiber: 5 g

Cooking Time: 1 hour

Serves: 6   **Rating:** ★★★★★

Shepherd's Pie is the ultimate comfort food, combining savory meat and vegetables under a layer of creamy mashed potatoes. Perfect for a hearty family dinner, it's a dish that warms from the inside out.

Pumpkin Pie

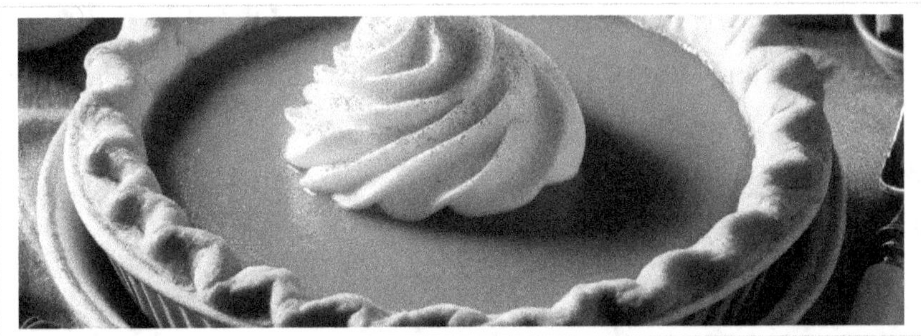

Ingredients:

- 1 (9-inch) unbaked pie crust
- 1 can (15 oz) pumpkin puree
- 3/4 cup sugar
- 1/2 teaspoon salt
- 1 teaspoon ground cinnamon
- 1/2 teaspoon ground ginger
- 1/4 teaspoon ground cloves
- 2 large eggs
- 1 can (12 oz) evaporated milk
- Whipped cream, for serving

Preparation:

1. Preheat your oven to 425°F (220°C).
2. In a large bowl, mix pumpkin puree, sugar, salt, cinnamon, ginger, and cloves.
3. Beat in eggs one at a time, then gradually stir in the evaporated milk.
4. Pour the mixture into the pie crust.
5. Bake for 15 minutes. Reduce the oven temperature to 350°F (175°C) and continue baking for 40-50 minutes, or until a knife inserted near the center comes out clean.
6. Cool on a wire rack. Serve with whipped cream, sprinkled with cinnamon or nutmeg if desired.

Nutritional Values:

- Calories: 280 kcal per slice
- Protein: 6 g
- Carbohydrates: 40 g
- Fat: 12 g
- Fiber: 2 g

Cooking Time: 1 hour 5 minutes

Serves: 8

Rating: ★★★★★

Pumpkin Pie is a hallmark of fall and holiday dining, celebrated for its creamy, spiced filling and flaky crust. This classic dessert offers a taste of nostalgia and warmth, perfect for ending a festive meal or enjoying as a comforting treat.

Chicken Pot Pie

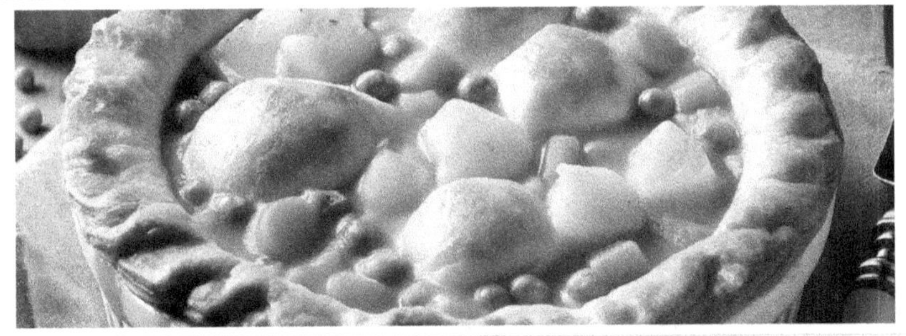

Ingredients:

- 1 lb chicken breast, cooked and diced
- 1 cup carrots, diced
- 1 cup frozen peas
- 1 cup diced potatoes
- 1/2 cup butter
- 1/2 cup chopped onion
- 1/3 cup all-purpose flour
- 1/2 teaspoon salt
- 1/4 teaspoon black pepper
- 1/4 teaspoon celery seed
- 1 3/4 cups chicken broth
- 2/3 cup milk
- 2 (9-inch) unbaked pie crusts

Preparation:

1. Preheat your oven to 425°F (220°C).
2. In a saucepan over medium heat, melt butter. Add onion, cook until translucent. Stir in flour, salt, pepper, and celery seed.
3. Slowly stir in chicken broth and milk. Simmer over medium-low heat until thick. Remove from heat, and mix in chicken, carrots, peas, and potatoes.

4. Place one crust in the bottom of a pie dish. Pour the chicken mixture into the crust. Cover with the second crust, seal edges, and cut away excess dough. Make several small slits in the top to allow steam to escape.

5. Bake for 30 to 35 minutes, or until pastry is golden brown and filling is bubbly. Cool for 10 minutes before serving.

Nutritional Values:

- Calories: 410 kcal per serving
- Protein: 20 g
- Carbohydrates: 35 g
- Fat: 20 g
- Fiber: 3 g

Cooking Time: 1 hour

Serves: 6

Rating: ★★★★★

Chicken Pot Pie is a classic comfort dish, featuring a creamy mixture of chicken and vegetables encased in a flaky pastry crust

Apple Pie

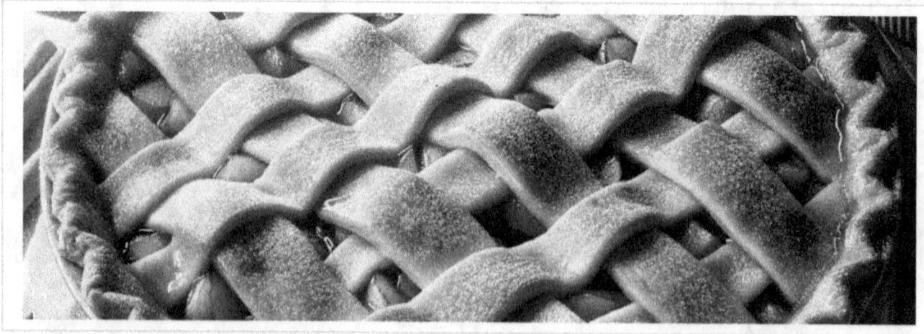

Ingredients:

- 2 pie crusts (for top and bottom)
- 6 cups thinly sliced apples (such as Granny Smith)
- 3/4 cup sugar
- 2 tablespoons all-purpose flour
- 1/2 teaspoon ground cinnamon
- 1/4 teaspoon ground nutmeg
- 1/4 teaspoon salt
- 2 tablespoons butter
- 1 egg yolk, beaten (for brushing)

Preparation:

1. Preheat your oven to 425°F (220°C).
2. Place one pie crust in a 9-inch pie dish. In a large bowl, toss the sliced apples with sugar, flour, cinnamon, nutmeg, and salt.
3. Pour the apple mixture into the crust-lined pie dish. Dot with pieces of butter.
4. Cover with the second crust. Trim excess dough, and crimp edges to seal. Cut slits in the top crust for steam to escape. Brush the top crust with beaten egg yolk.
5. Bake in the preheated oven for 15 minutes. Reduce the temperature to 350°F (175°C) and continue baking for another 35-45 minutes, or until the crust is golden and the filling is bubbly.
6. Allow to cool before serving. Serve with a scoop of vanilla ice cream, if desired.

Nutritional Values:

- Calories: 330 kcal per slice
- Protein: 3 g
- Carbohydrates: 50 g
- Fat: 14 g
- Fiber: 3 g

Cooking Time: 1 hour

Serves: 8

Rating: ★★★★★

Apple Pie is a timeless dessert that captures the essence of home and comfort with its spiced apple filling and flaky crust. Whether served at a family gathering or as a sweet treat, it's a beloved classic that never fails to delight.

Pecan Pie

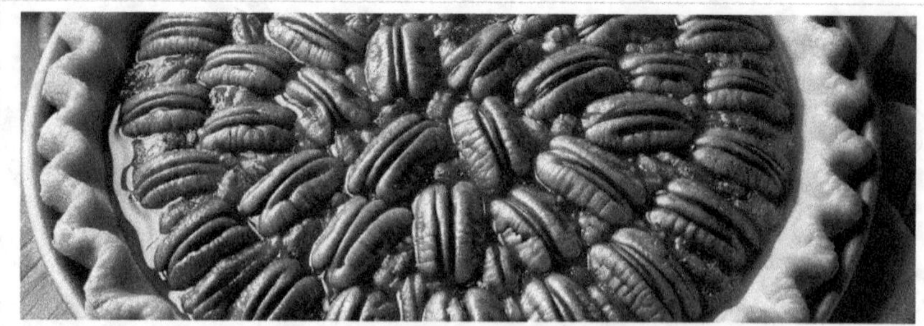

Ingredients:

- 1 pie crust (9-inch, unbaked)
- 1 cup light corn syrup
- 1 cup brown sugar
- 3 eggs, beaten
- 1/3 cup butter, melted
- 1 teaspoon vanilla extract
- 1 1/2 cups pecan halves

Preparation:

1. Preheat your oven to 350°F (175°C).
2. In a large bowl, mix corn syrup, brown sugar, eggs, butter, and vanilla until smooth. Stir in pecan halves.
3. Pour the filling into the unbaked pie crust.
4. Bake for 60 to 70 minutes, or until the filling is set and the pie is golden brown. The center should slightly jiggle when shaken.
5. Cool on a wire rack before serving.

Nutritional Values:

- Calories: 510 kcal per slice
- Protein: 6 g
- Carbohydrates: 65 g
- Fat: 28 g
- Fiber: 2 g

Cooking Time: 1 hour 10 minutes

Serves: 8

Rating: ★★★★★

Pecan Pie is a decadent dessert that combines the crunchiness of pecans with a sweet, caramel-like filling, all encased in a flaky crust. It's a beloved treat for special occasions and holidays, offering a rich and satisfying end to any meal.

APPENDICES

Tips for Grocery Shopping and Meal Prepping

Navigating the grocery store and meal prepping can seem daunting at first, but with a few strategic tips, you'll be on your way to becoming a pro in no time. Here's how to make your grocery shopping and meal prepping both efficient and enjoyable:

1. **Make a Plan:** Before you even step foot in the store, know what you're shopping for. Create a weekly meal plan and list all the ingredients you need. This not only saves time but also helps prevent impulse buys.

2. **Shop the Perimeter:** The freshest foods like fruits, vegetables, dairy, and meats are typically located around the store's perimeter. Start there to fill your cart with whole foods, then move inward for other essentials.

3. **Buy in Bulk:** For non-perishable items or foods you use often, buying in bulk can save money. Just make sure you have the storage space and that these items won't go to waste.

4. **Choose Whole Foods:** Whenever possible, pick whole foods over processed ones. Whole grains, lean meats, and fresh produce are more nutritious and often more satisfying.

5. **Prep Right Away:** When you get home from the store, take some time to wash, chop, and store fruits and vegetables. You can also cook grains or proteins ahead of time. This makes putting meals together during the week much faster.

6. **Invest in Good Containers:** Having a variety of sizes for storage containers can make meal prepping easier. Look for microwave-safe and freezer-friendly options to expand your meal storage solutions.

7. **Keep It Simple:** Meal prepping doesn't have to mean cooking all your meals in advance. It can be as simple as prepping ingredients to mix and match for quick assembly during the week.

8. **Be Flexible:** Sometimes, the avocados you planned to buy aren't ripe, or the salmon is too pricey. Be willing to adapt your meal plan based on what looks good and what's on sale.

9. **Portion Control:** If you're meal prepping for health reasons, pay attention to portion sizes as you prep. This makes it easier to grab-and-go without overeating.

10. **Have Fun with It:** Experiment with new recipes or ingredients each week to keep things interesting. Cooking and meal prepping should be enjoyable, not a chore.

Remember, the goal of grocery shopping and meal prepping is to make your life easier and healthier. Don't stress about getting it perfect. Over time, you'll find what strategies work best for you and your lifestyle. Happy prepping!

Meal Planning Templates

These templates are designed to offer variety and balance throughout the week/month, incorporating dishes from different chapters to ensure a mix of flavors and nutrients.

Weekly Meal Plan

Monday:

- Breakfast: Sunrise Smoothie

- Lunch: Kale and Quinoa Salad

- Dinner: Grilled Salmon with Asparagus

- Snack: Almond Butter Cups

Tuesday:

- Breakfast: Avocado Toast with Poached Egg

- Lunch: Turkey Avocado Wraps

- Dinner: Spaghetti Squash with Marinara Sauce

- Snack: Carrot Cake Energy Balls

Wednesday:

- Breakfast: Quinoa Porridge with Berries

- Lunch: Broccoli and Chickpea Bowl

- Dinner: Beef Stir-Fry with Broccoli

- Snack: Coconut Flour Cookies

Thursday:

- Breakfast: Spinach and Mushroom Omelette

- Lunch: Grilled Chicken Salad

- Dinner: Chicken and Vegetable Skewers

- Snack: Baked Apple Chips

Friday:

- Breakfast: Chia Seed Pudding

- Lunch: Butternut Squash Soup

- Dinner: Lamb Stew

- Snack: Avocado Chocolate Mousse

Saturday:

- Breakfast: Banana Almond Smoothie

- Lunch: Leftovers or your choice

- Dinner: Pork Chops with Peach Salsa

- Snack: Your choice

Sunday:

- Breakfast: Coconut Yogurt Parfait

- Lunch: Mixed Greens with Avocado

- Dinner: Slow-Cooked Beef Ragu

- Snack: Your choice

Monthly Meal Plan (Sample Week)

Week 1: Refer to the weekly plan above.

Week 2:

- Breakfasts: Alternate between Sweet Potato Hash and Apple Cinnamon Oatmeal

- Lunches: Rotate Kale and Quinoa Salad, Shrimp and Avocado Salad, and Chicken Pesto Pizza

- Dinners: Choose from Grilled Tuna Steaks, Beef Kabobs, and Zucchini Lasagna

- Snacks: Try Almond Butter Cups and Baked Apple Chips

Week 3:

- Breakfasts: Mix it up with Berry Bliss Smoothie and Avocado Toast with Poached Egg

- Lunches: Enjoy leftovers, Cauliflower Crust Margherita Pizza, and Spinach and Goat Cheese Pizza

- Dinners: Prepare Eggplant Parmesan Casserole, Chicken Pot Pie, and Pan-Seared Scallops

- Snacks: Savor Carrot Cake Energy Balls and Avocado Chocolate Mousse

Week 4:

- Breakfasts: Go for Chia Seed Pudding and Quinoa Porridge with Berries

- Lunches: Have Lentil and Sweet Potato Stew, Beef and Broccoli, and BBQ Chicken Pizza

- Dinners: Choose from Pork Tenderloin with Apples, Shepherd's Pie, and Pumpkin Pie (for a treat)

- Snacks: Enjoy Coconut Flour Cookies and Almond Butter Cups

This template is a guide to help you start meal planning with the recipes provided. Feel free to adjust the meals to fit your schedule, dietary preferences, and nutritional needs. Enjoy exploring the flavors and benefits of home-cooked meals!

Shopping Lists

Produce:

- Avocados
- Mixed berries (strawberries, blueberries, raspberries)
- Spinach
- Mushrooms
- Apples
- Sweet potatoes
- Zucchini
- Broccoli
- Carrots
- Peas
- Onions (red, white)
- Garlic
- Lemons
- Limes
- Tomatoes (cherry, whole)
- Basil, cilantro, parsley, rosemary, thyme
- Kale
- Arugula
- Cucumbers
- Lettuce
- Cauliflower
- Brussels sprouts
- Green beans

- Potatoes

Protein:

- Chicken (breast, whole)

- Ground lamb or beef

- Tuna (canned and fresh)

- Salmon (fillets)

- Cod

- Shrimp

- Eggs

- Pork (tenderloin, chops)

Dairy:

- Milk (dairy and almond)

- Mozzarella cheese

- Parmesan cheese

- Cheddar cheese

- Ricotta cheese

- Sour cream

- Butter

- Goat cheese

- Yogurt (plain, coconut)

Pantry Items:

- Olive oil

- Coconut oil

- Balsamic vinegar

- Soy sauce

- Tomato paste

- Marinara sauce

- Chicken broth

- Beef broth

- Canned chickpeas

- Canned pumpkin

- Canned crushed tomatoes

- Evaporated milk

- Corn syrup

- Brown sugar

- Sugar

- Honey

- Maple syrup

- Vanilla extract

- Breadcrumbs

- Crackers

- Nuts (pecans, almonds, walnuts)

- Seeds (chia seeds)

- Dark chocolate/chocolate chips

- Cocoa powder

- Coconut flour

- All-purpose flour

- Pie crusts

- Panko breadcrumbs

- Quinoa

- Lentils

- Pasta (regular and egg noodles)

- Rice

Spices & Herbs:

- Salt & pepper

- Cinnamon

- Nutmeg

- Ground ginger

- Ground cloves

- Celery seed

- Garlic powder

- Red pepper flakes

Frozen:

- Frozen peas

- Frozen corn

This list aims to equip you with the majority of ingredients needed for the recipes in this cookbook. Remember, fresh is best, but don't hesitate to use frozen or canned versions of fruits and vegetables to save time and money. Adjust the list based on your meal plan, dietary preferences, and the number of servings you need. Happy cooking and shopping!

Substitution Chart for Common Ingredients

Creating a substitution chart for common ingredients can be a lifesaver in the kitchen, especially when you're in the middle of a recipe and realize you're missing an ingredient. Here's a handy chart to help you navigate those moments without a hitch.

Dairy Substitutes

- **Milk:** For 1 cup of milk, use 1 cup of soy, almond, or oat milk.

- **Buttermilk:** Mix 1 cup of milk (or a dairy-free alternative) with 1 tablespoon of lemon juice or white vinegar; let sit for 5 minutes.

- **Heavy Cream:** For 1 cup of heavy cream, use 1 cup of coconut cream or 3/4 cup milk mixed with 1/4 cup melted butter.

- **Sour Cream/Yogurt:** Use 1 cup of plain Greek yogurt or dairy-free yogurt.

Sugar Substitutes

- **White Sugar:** For 1 cup of sugar, use 1 cup of honey, maple syrup, or agave nectar (reduce the liquid in the recipe by 3 tablespoons).

- **Brown Sugar:** Use 1 cup white sugar plus 1 tablespoon molasses.

Fat Substitutes

- **Butter:** For 1 cup of butter, use 1 cup of margarine, coconut oil, or applesauce (for baking).

- **Oil:** For baking, use equal amounts of applesauce or mashed bananas to replace oil.

Egg Substitutes (in baking)

- **1 Egg:** Use 1/4 cup of applesauce, mashed banana, or 1 tablespoon of ground flaxseed mixed with 3 tablespoons of water.

Flour Substitutes

- **All-Purpose Flour:** For 1 cup of flour, use 1 cup of whole wheat flour, or for gluten-free options, use 1 cup of almond flour or oat flour (note that the texture might change).

- **Bread Crumbs:** Use 3/4 cup of rolled oats or crumbled crackers.

Meat Substitutes

- **Ground Beef:** Use equal amounts of ground turkey, chicken, or for a vegetarian option, cooked and mashed lentils or a meat substitute like Beyond Meat.

Chocolate Substitutes

- **Cocoa Powder:** For every 3 tablespoons of cocoa powder, use 1 ounce of unsweetened chocolate, adjusting the recipe's sugar accordingly.

- **Chocolate Chips:** Use an equal amount of chopped chocolate bars, noting the cocoa content for sweetness.

Miscellaneous

- **Lemon Juice:** For 1 tablespoon of lemon juice, use 1/2 tablespoon of white vinegar or lime juice.

- **Wine in Cooking:** Use chicken or vegetable broth, or for sweetness, use apple juice or white grape juice.

Remember, while substitutions can be incredibly helpful, they may slightly alter the taste, texture, or appearance of your dish. It's all part of the adventure in cooking! Experiment and see what works best for your recipes and preferences.

Thank You

I'm writing this with a heart full of gratitude for your kind words and the time you took to read my book, knowing that my words have resonated with you is a reward beyond measure. Thank you again for your appreciation and for being a part of this literary journey.

Warmly,

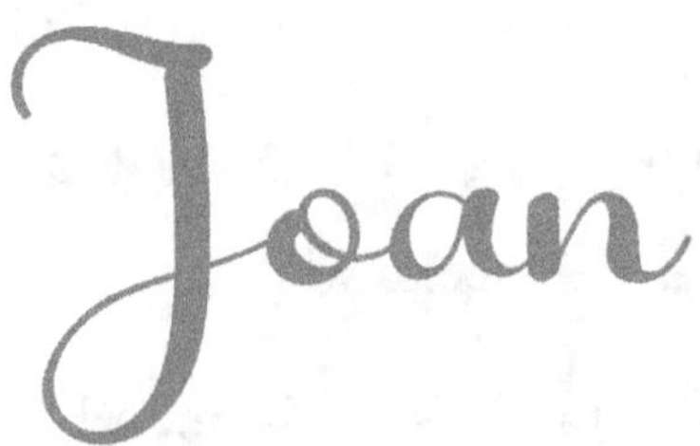

Joan

For further Questions and advice reach out on

joanmilonehelpdesk@gmail.com

Your voice matters to us! Dive into the pages of our latest book and embark on a journey of discovery, adventure, and insight. Once you've turned the last page, we invite you to share your thoughts with us.

Your honest review is incredibly important for several reasons: It not only helps us grow and improve by understanding what resonates with our readers, but it also assists fellow readers in making informed decisions about their next reading choice. In a way, your feedback lights the path for future stories and enriches our reading community. So, take a moment, reflect on your journey through our story, and leave a review that could light the way for others. Together, let's create a community of passionate readers and insightful feedback.

Thank you for being a part of our story – we can't wait to hear from you!

Kindly open your phone camera and place it on the barcode to scan

It will link you directly to author page to access more cookbooks from us

Very seamless…

30 Days

Meal

Planner

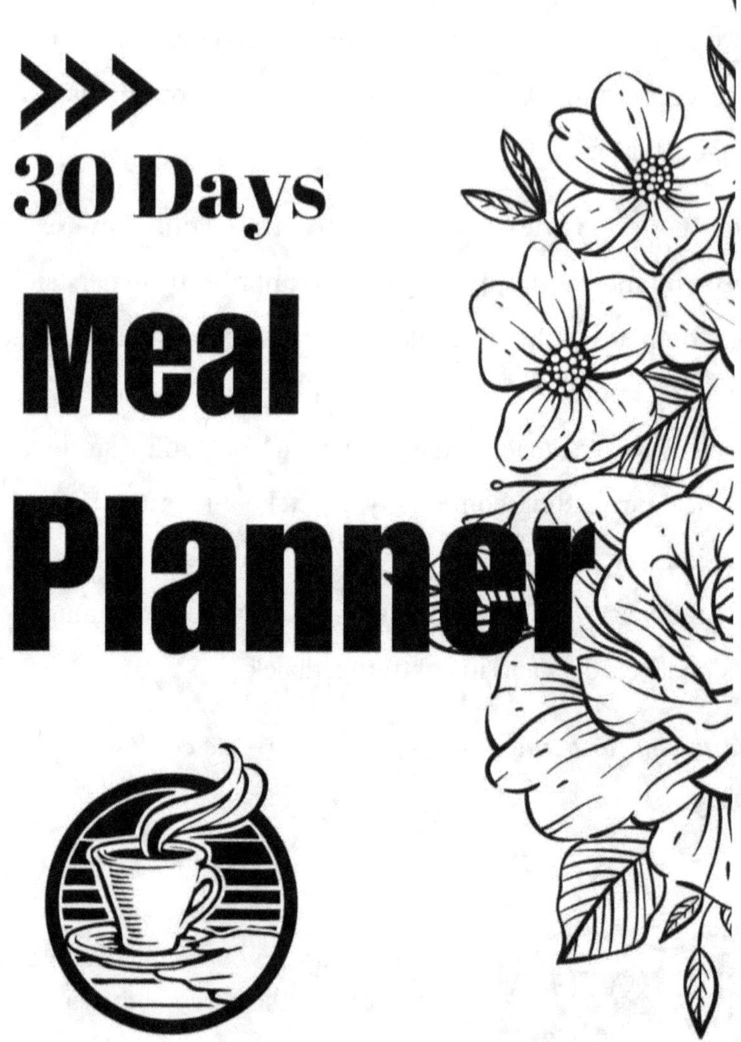

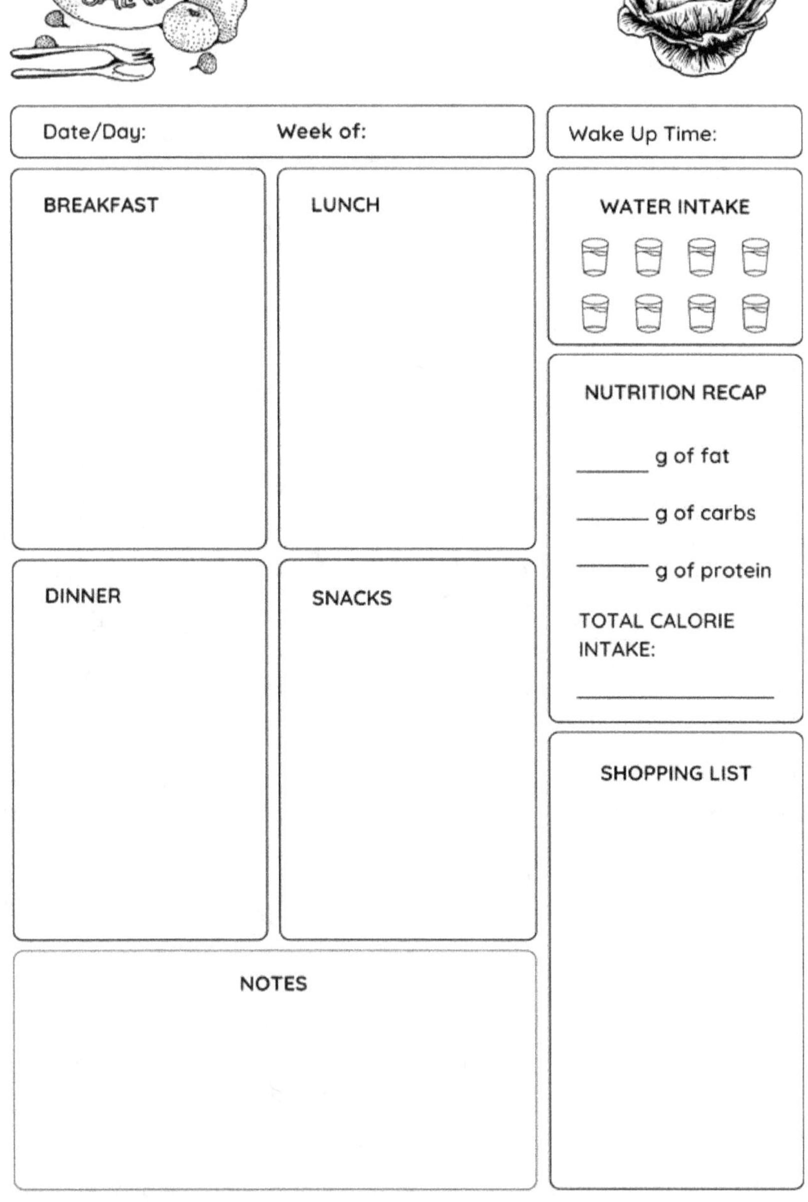

Date/Day: Week of:

Wake Up Time:

BREAKFAST

LUNCH

WATER INTAKE

NUTRITION RECAP

_______ g of fat

_______ g of carbs

_______ g of protein

TOTAL CALORIE
INTAKE:

____

DINNER

SNACKS

SHOPPING LIST

NOTES

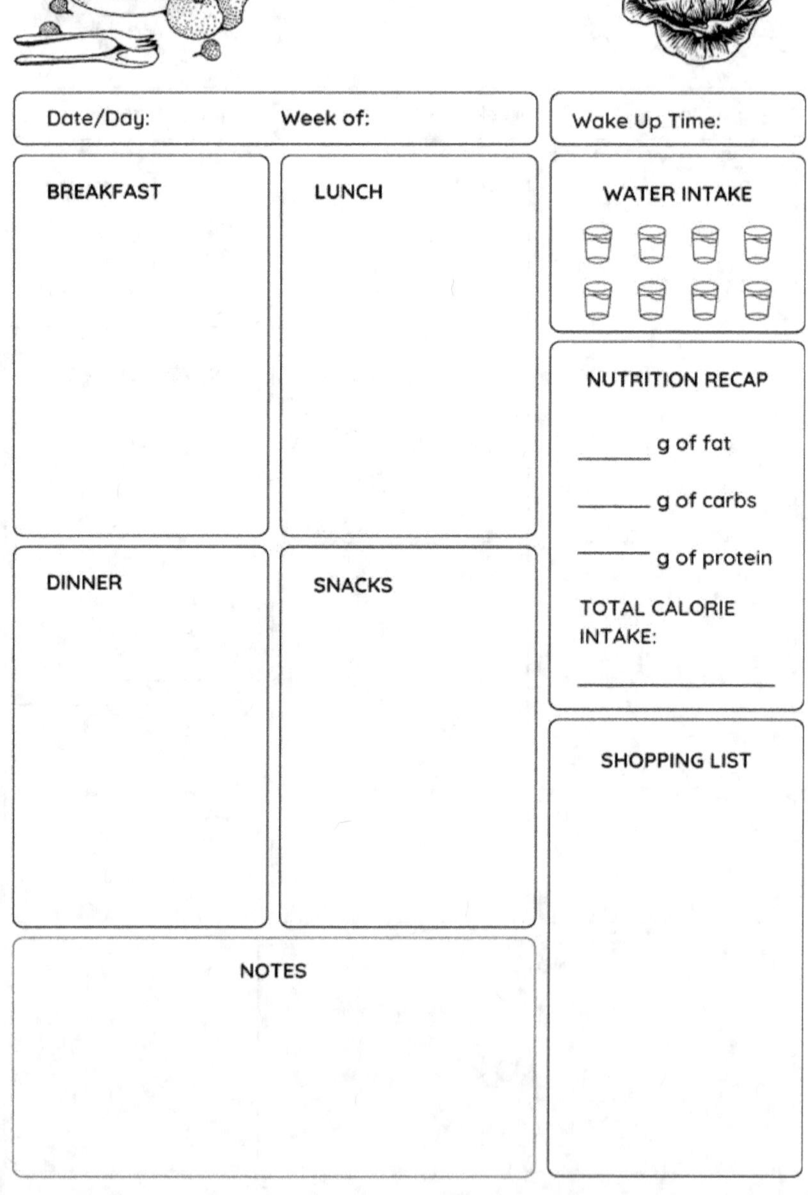
SALAD
Date/Day:
Week of:
Wake Up Time:
BREAKFAST
LUNCH
WATER INTAKE
NUTRITION RECAP
______ g of fat
______ g of carbs
______ g of protein
TOTAL CALORIE
INTAKE:
DINNER
SNACKS
SHOPPING LIST
NOTES

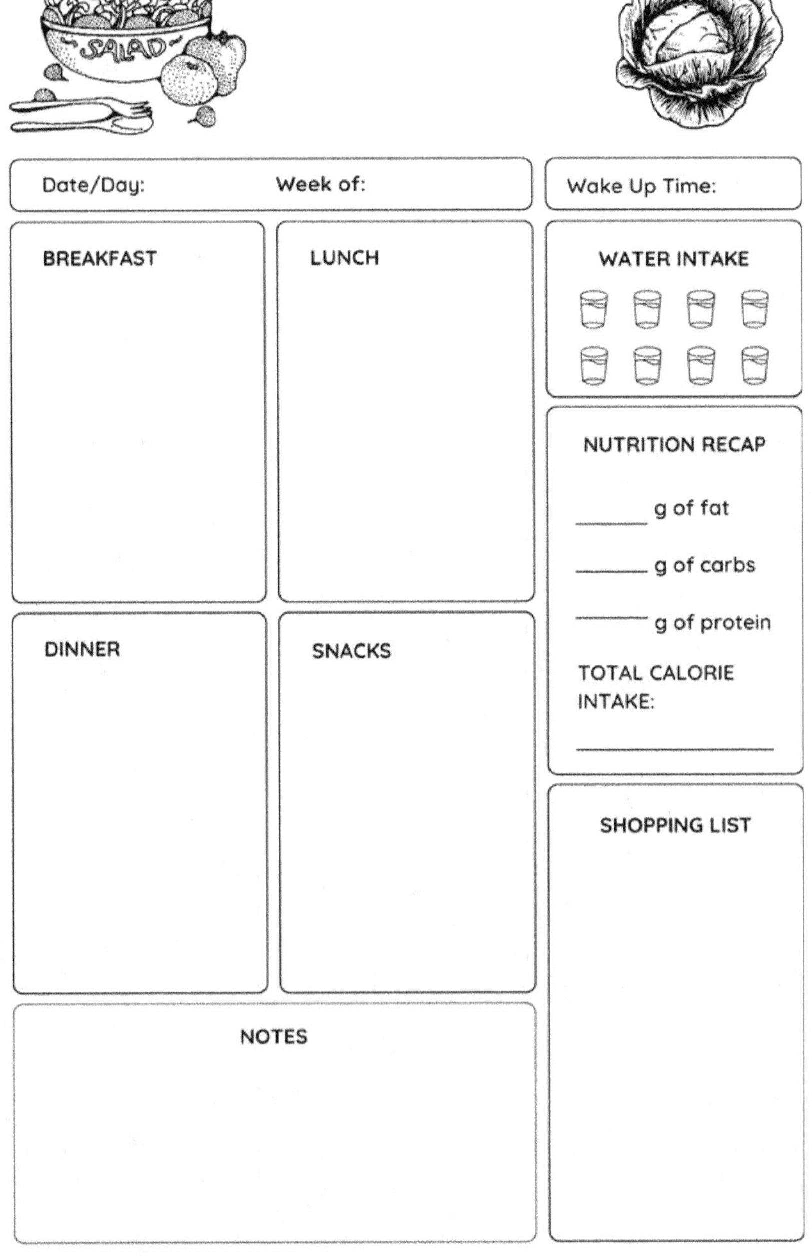

| Date/Day: | Week of: | Wake Up Time: |

BREAKFAST

LUNCH

WATER INTAKE

DINNER

SNACKS

NUTRITION RECAP

________ g of fat

________ g of carbs

________ g of protein

TOTAL CALORIE INTAKE:

SHOPPING LIST

NOTES

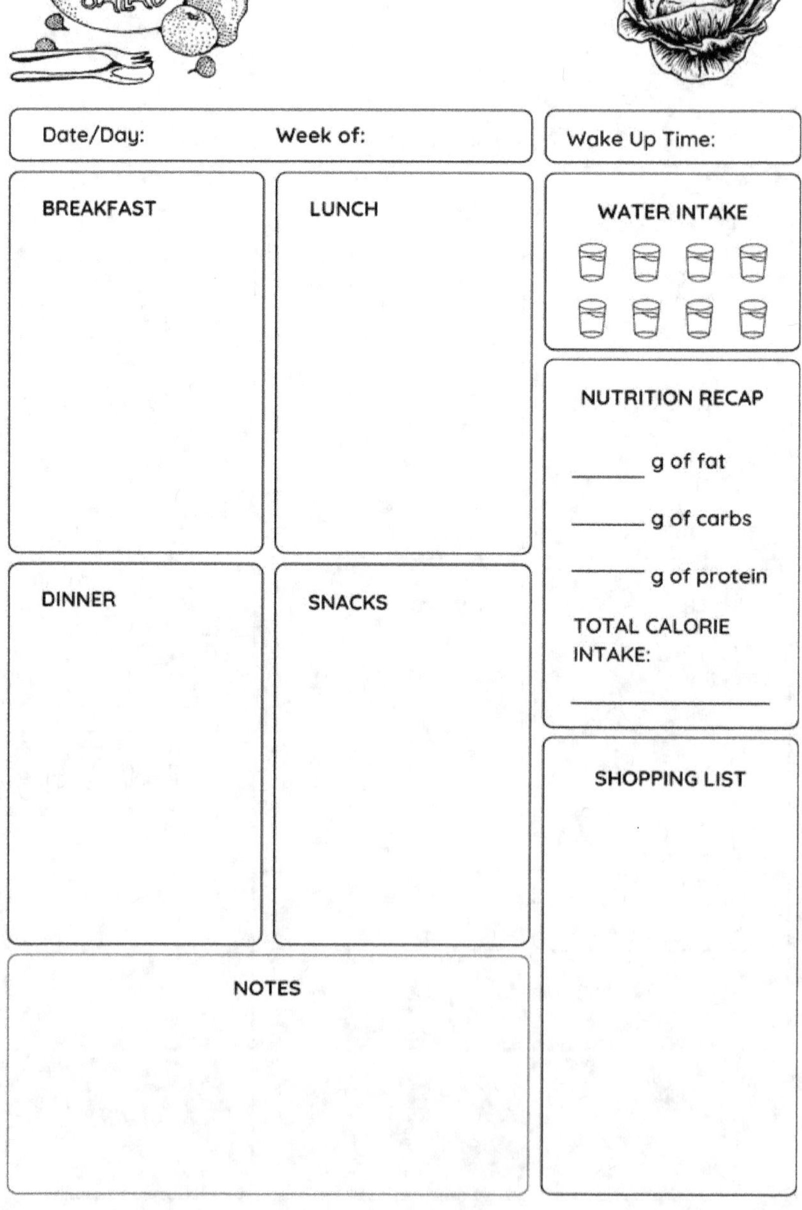

| Date/Day: | Week of: | Wake Up Time: |

BREAKFAST

LUNCH

WATER INTAKE

NUTRITION RECAP

_______ g of fat

_______ g of carbs

_______ g of protein

TOTAL CALORIE INTAKE:

DINNER

SNACKS

SHOPPING LIST

NOTES

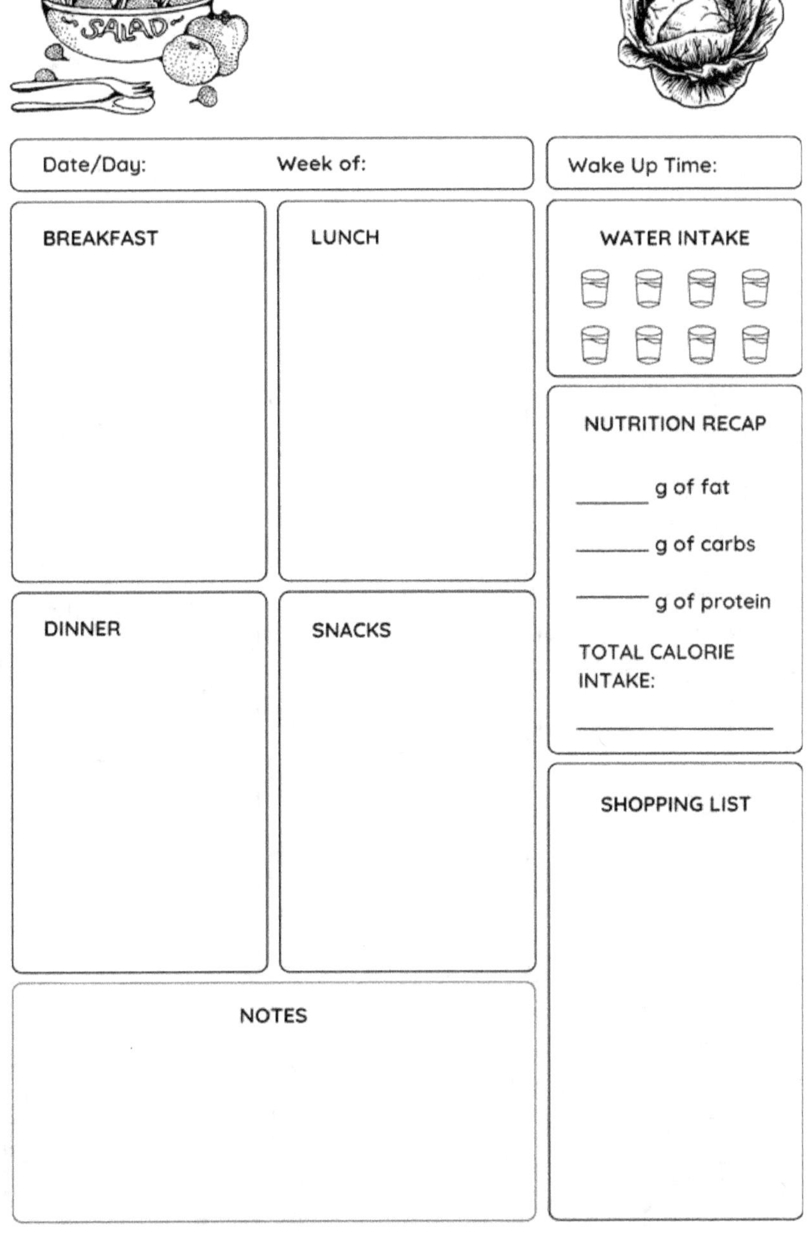

| Date/Day: | Week of: | Wake Up Time: |

BREAKFAST

LUNCH

WATER INTAKE

NUTRITION RECAP

_______ g of fat

_______ g of carbs

_______ g of protein

TOTAL CALORIE INTAKE:

____

DINNER

SNACKS

SHOPPING LIST

NOTES

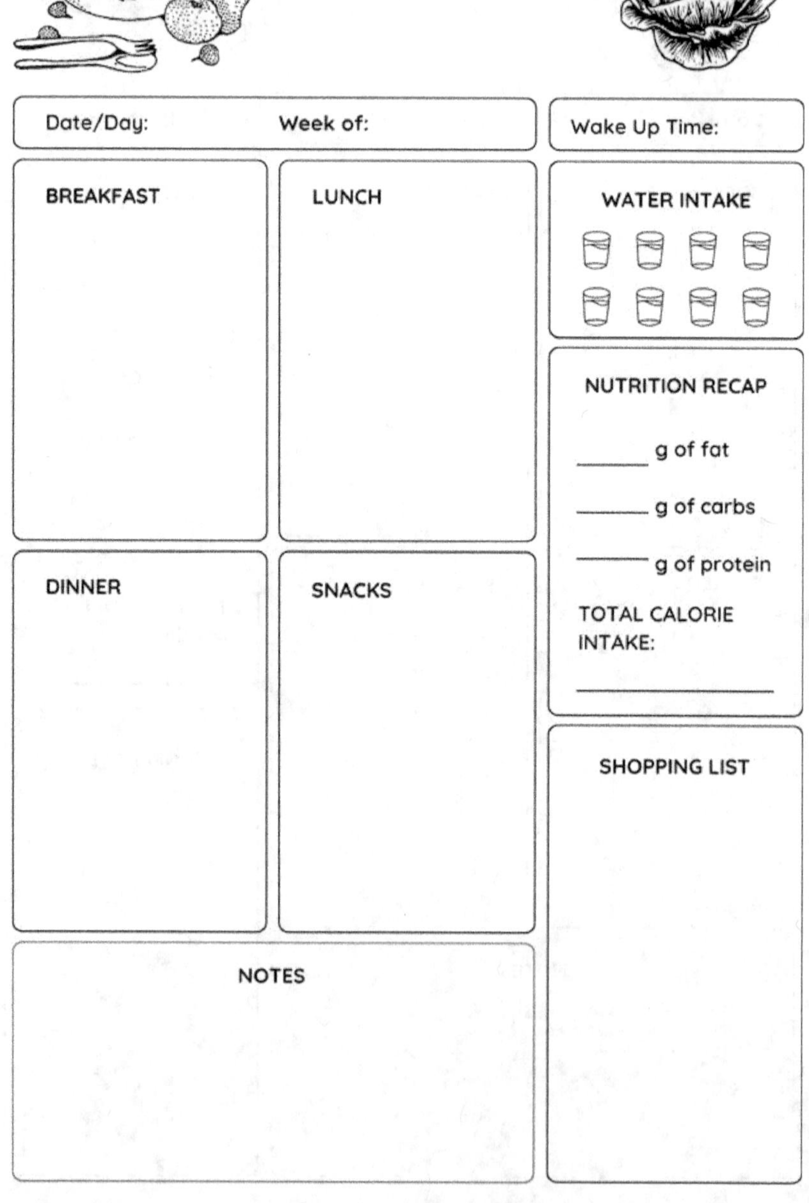

Date/Day: Week of:

Wake Up Time:

BREAKFAST

LUNCH

WATER INTAKE

NUTRITION RECAP

_______ g of fat

_______ g of carbs

_______ g of protein

TOTAL CALORIE
INTAKE:

____

DINNER

SNACKS

SHOPPING LIST

NOTES

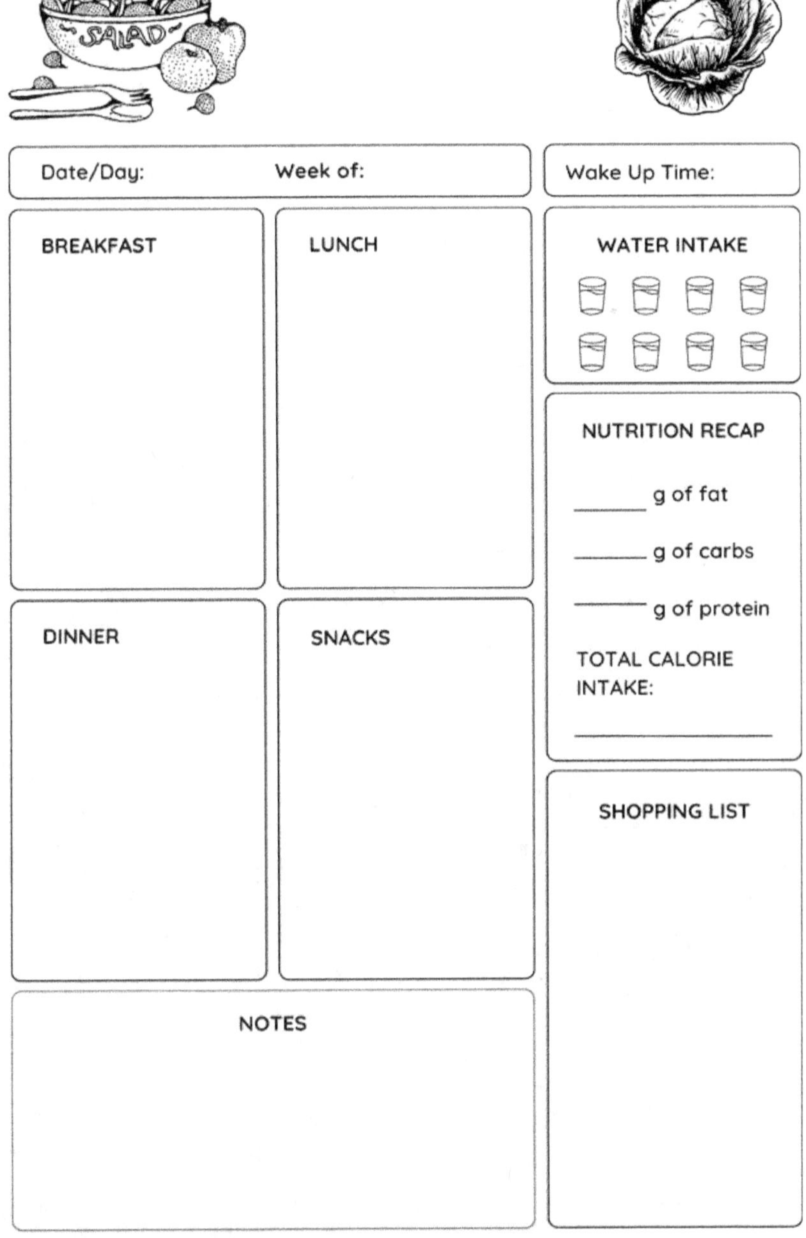

| Date/Day: | Week of: | Wake Up Time: |

BREAKFAST

LUNCH

WATER INTAKE

NUTRITION RECAP

_________ g of fat

_________ g of carbs

_________ g of protein

TOTAL CALORIE INTAKE:

____

DINNER

SNACKS

SHOPPING LIST

NOTES

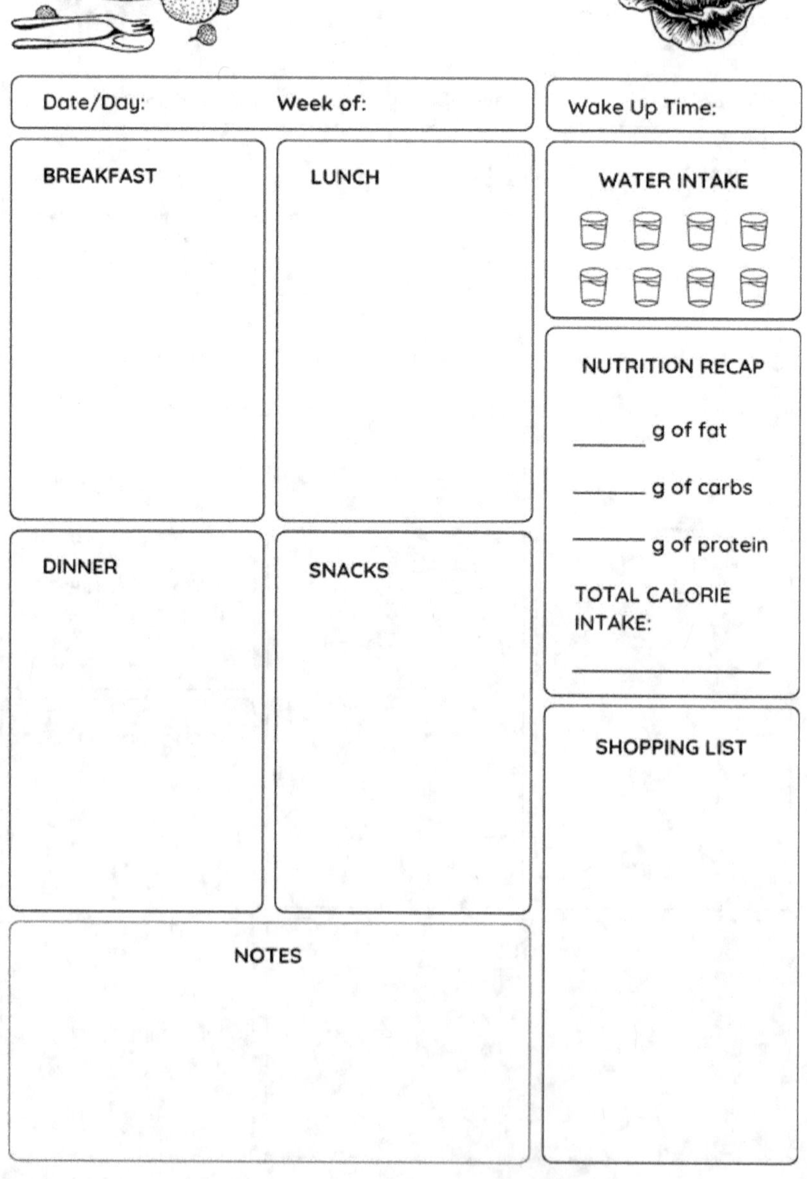

Date/Day:	Week of:		Wake Up Time:

BREAKFAST

LUNCH

WATER INTAKE

NUTRITION RECAP

_______ g of fat

_______ g of carbs

_______ g of protein

TOTAL CALORIE INTAKE:

____

DINNER

SNACKS

SHOPPING LIST

NOTES

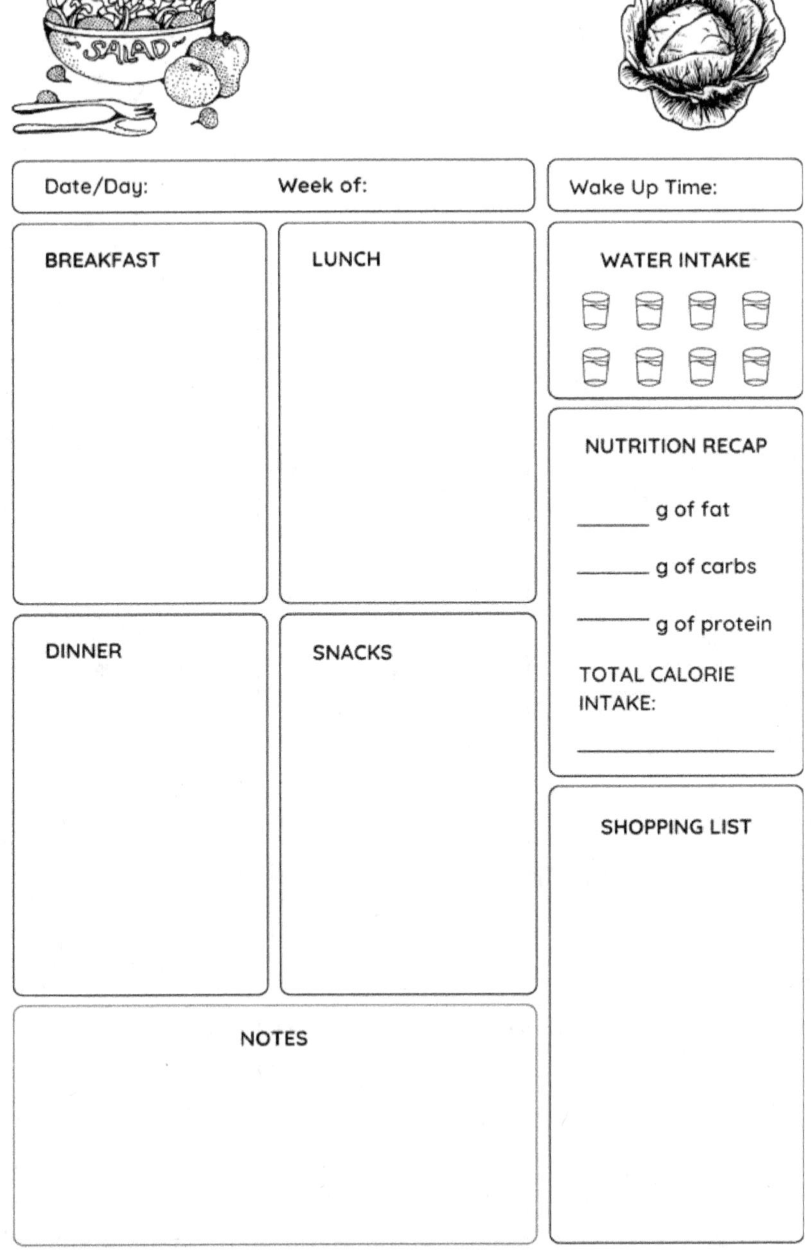

Date/Day: Week of:

Wake Up Time:

BREAKFAST

LUNCH

WATER INTAKE

NUTRITION RECAP

_______ g of fat

_______ g of carbs

_______ g of protein

TOTAL CALORIE INTAKE:

____

DINNER

SNACKS

SHOPPING LIST

NOTES

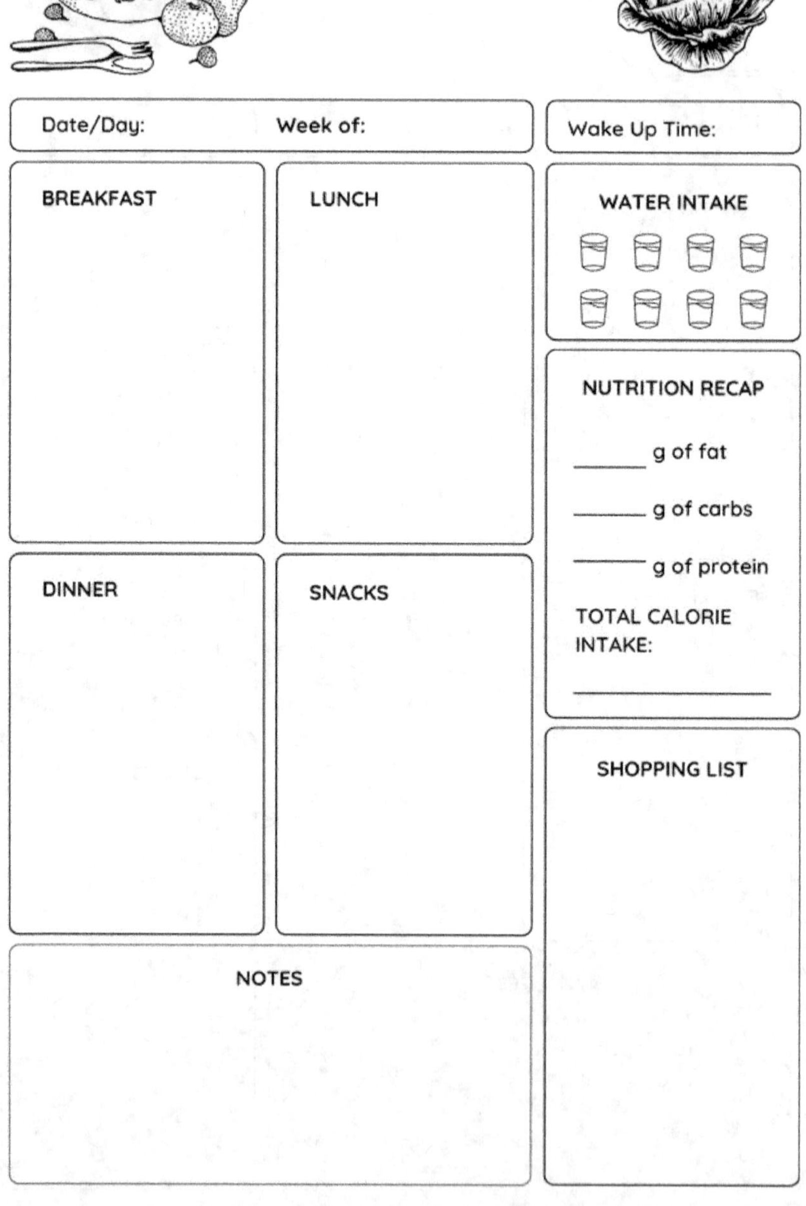

| Date/Day: | Week of: | Wake Up Time: |

BREAKFAST

LUNCH

WATER INTAKE

NUTRITION RECAP

_______ g of fat

_______ g of carbs

_______ g of protein

TOTAL CALORIE INTAKE:

____

DINNER

SNACKS

SHOPPING LIST

NOTES

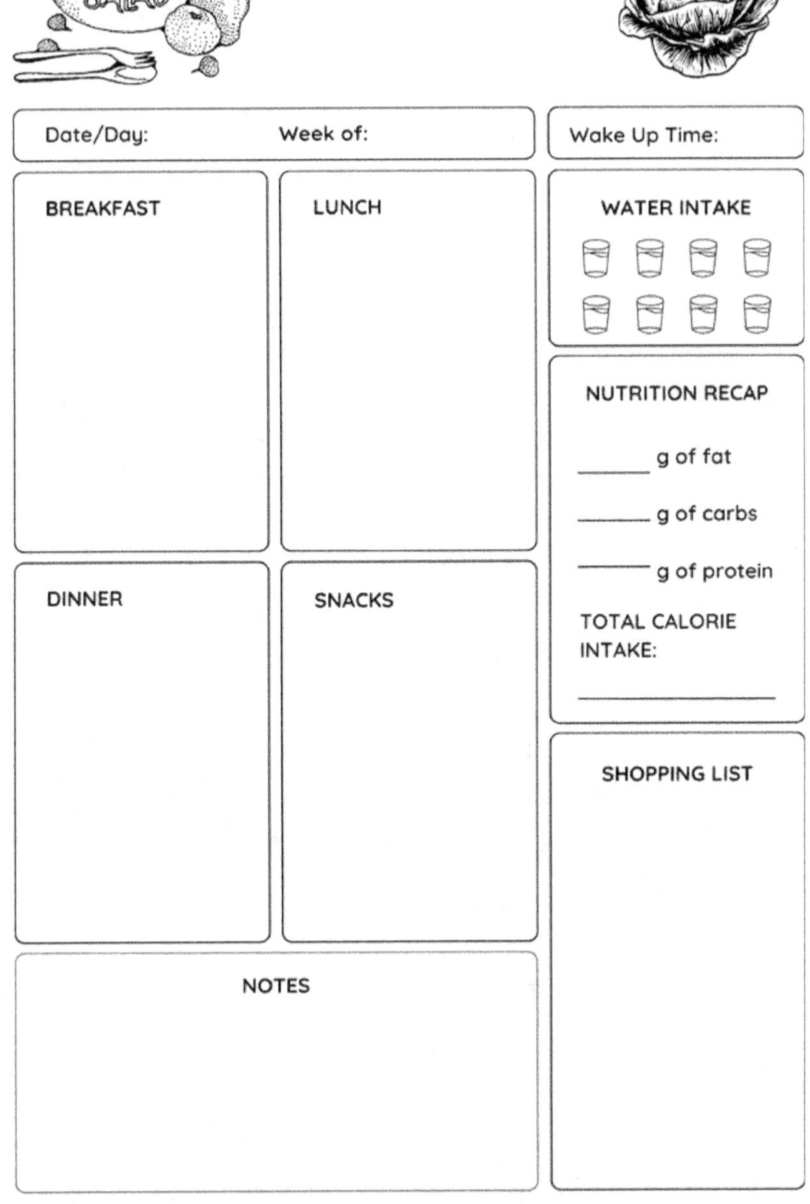

Date/Day: Week of:

Wake Up Time:

BREAKFAST

LUNCH

WATER INTAKE

NUTRITION RECAP

_______ g of fat

_______ g of carbs

_______ g of protein

TOTAL CALORIE INTAKE:

____

DINNER

SNACKS

SHOPPING LIST

NOTES

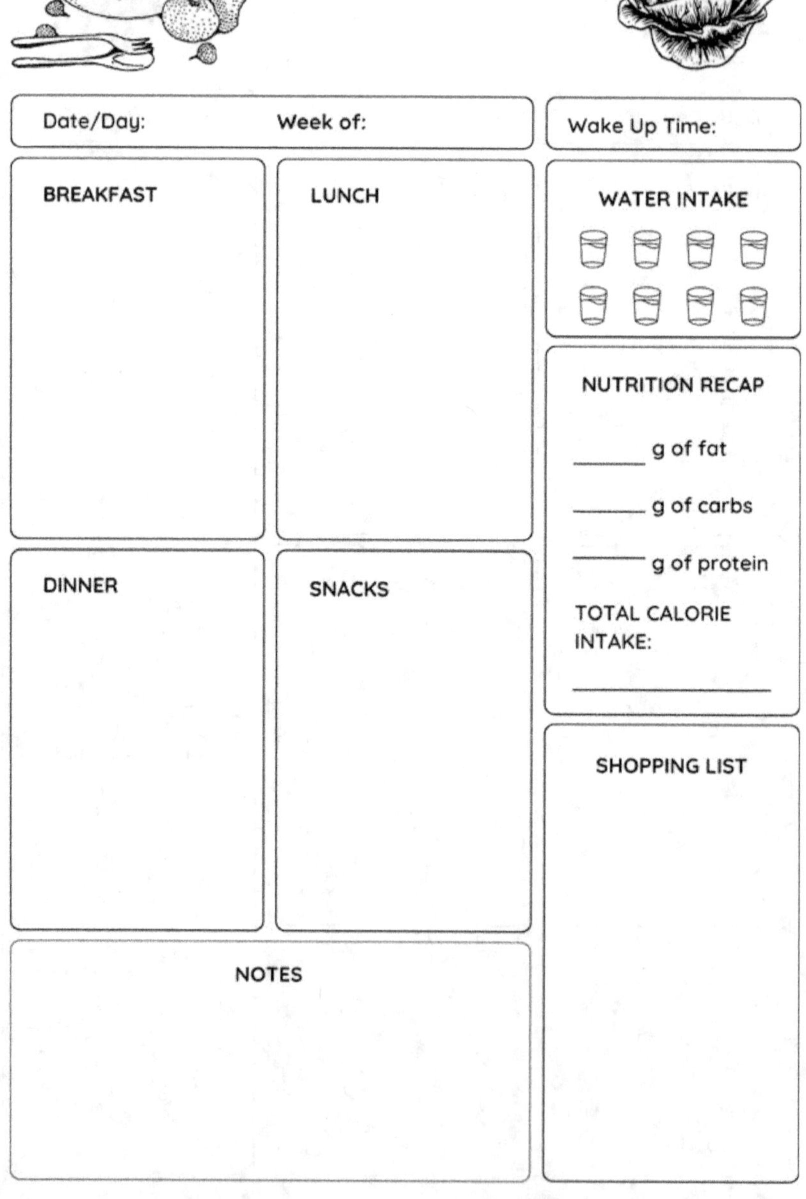
Date/Day:
Week of:
Wake Up Time:
BREAKFAST
LUNCH
WATER INTAKE
NUTRITION RECAP
________ g of fat
________ g of carbs
________ g of protein
TOTAL CALORIE
INTAKE:
DINNER
SNACKS
SHOPPING LIST
NOTES

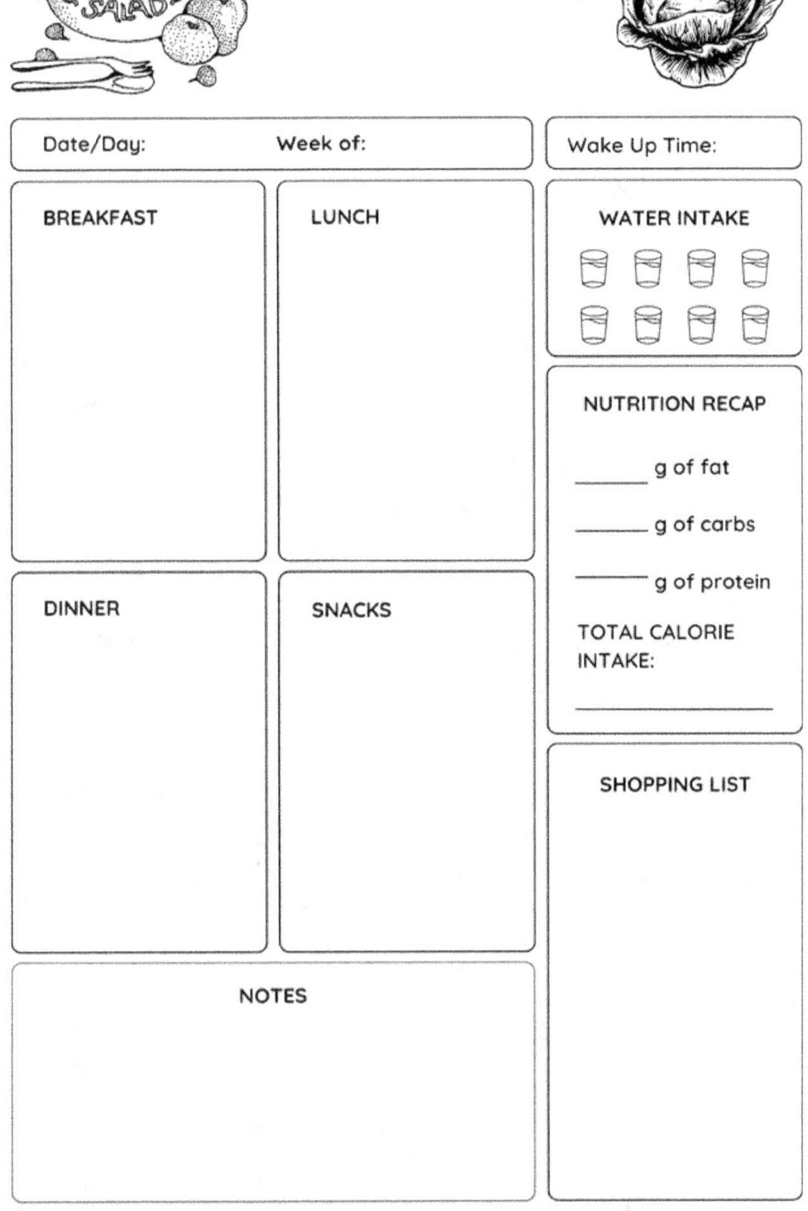

Date/Day: Week of:

Wake Up Time:

BREAKFAST

LUNCH

WATER INTAKE

NUTRITION RECAP

_______ g of fat

_______ g of carbs

_______ g of protein

TOTAL CALORIE INTAKE:

____

DINNER

SNACKS

SHOPPING LIST

NOTES

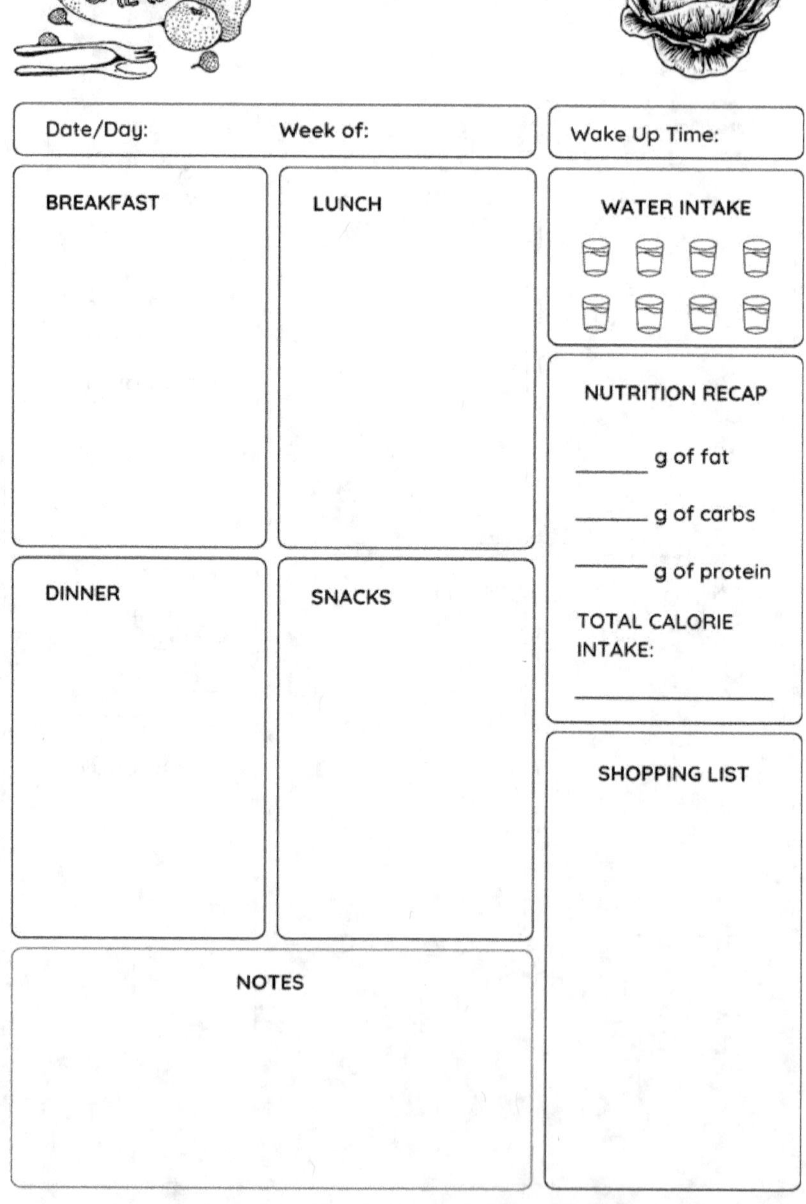

| Date/Day: | Week of: | Wake Up Time: |

BREAKFAST

LUNCH

WATER INTAKE

NUTRITION RECAP

_______ g of fat

_______ g of carbs

_______ g of protein

DINNER

SNACKS

TOTAL CALORIE INTAKE:

____

SHOPPING LIST

NOTES

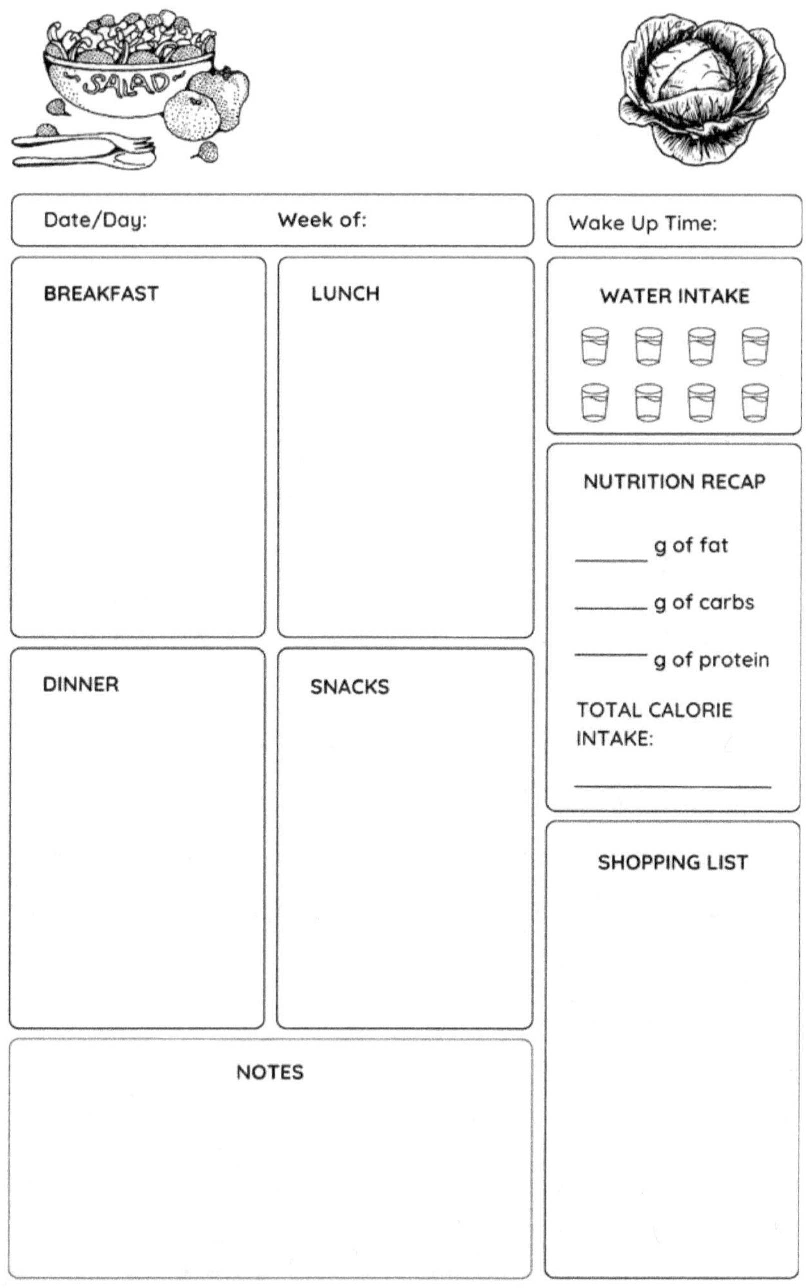

Date/Day: Week of:

Wake Up Time:

BREAKFAST

LUNCH

WATER INTAKE

NUTRITION RECAP

_______ g of fat

_______ g of carbs

_______ g of protein

TOTAL CALORIE INTAKE:

____

DINNER

SNACKS

SHOPPING LIST

NOTES

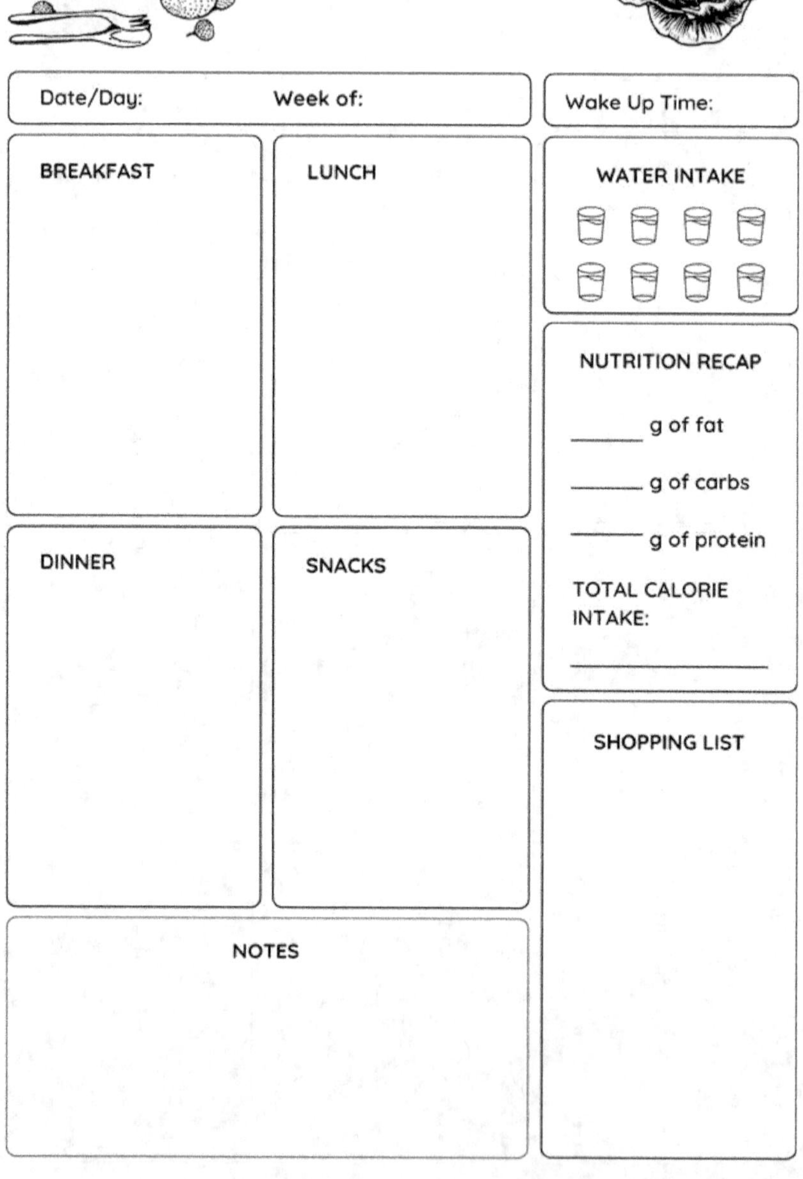

| Date/Day: | Week of: | Wake Up Time: |

BREAKFAST

LUNCH

WATER INTAKE

NUTRITION RECAP

_________ g of fat

_________ g of carbs

_________ g of protein

TOTAL CALORIE INTAKE:

____

DINNER

SNACKS

SHOPPING LIST

NOTES

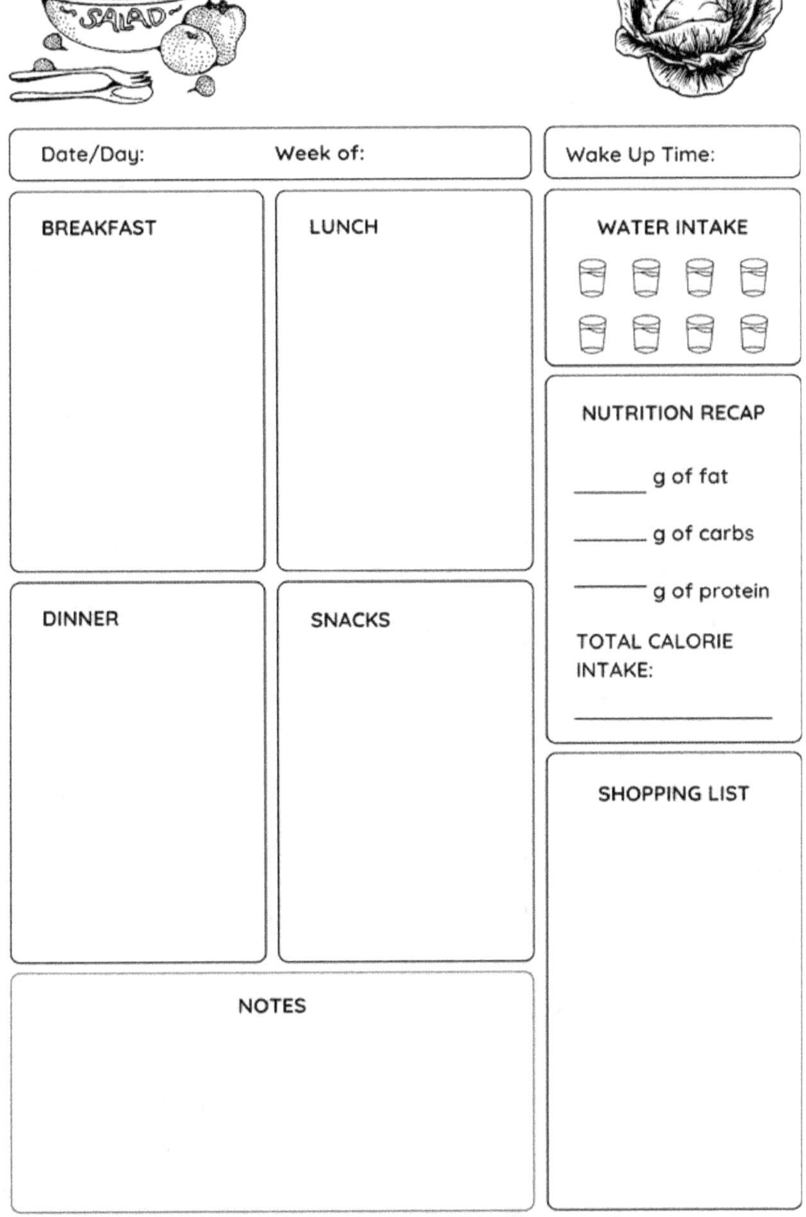

Date/Day: Week of:

Wake Up Time:

BREAKFAST

LUNCH

WATER INTAKE

NUTRITION RECAP

________ g of fat

________ g of carbs

________ g of protein

TOTAL CALORIE INTAKE:

____

DINNER

SNACKS

SHOPPING LIST

NOTES

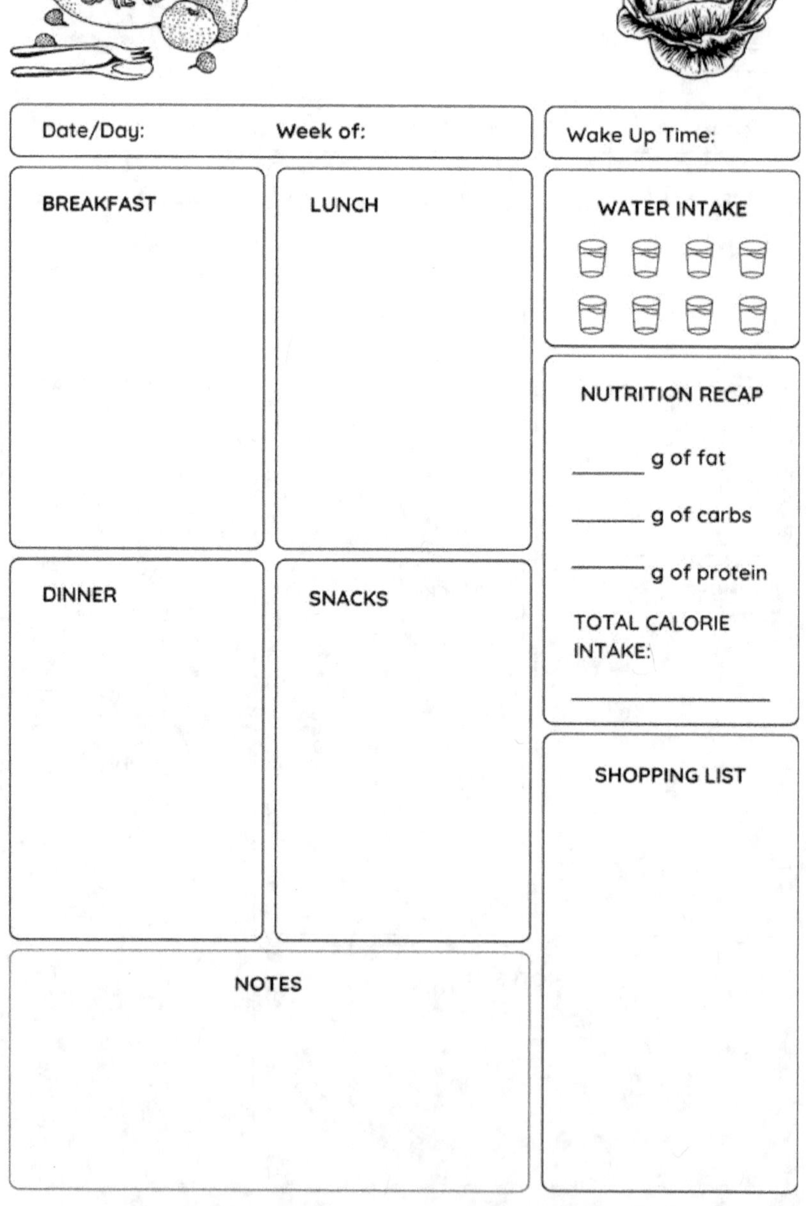

| Date/Day: | Week of: | Wake Up Time: |

BREAKFAST

LUNCH

WATER INTAKE

NUTRITION RECAP

_______ g of fat

_______ g of carbs

_______ g of protein

TOTAL CALORIE INTAKE:

____

DINNER

SNACKS

SHOPPING LIST

NOTES

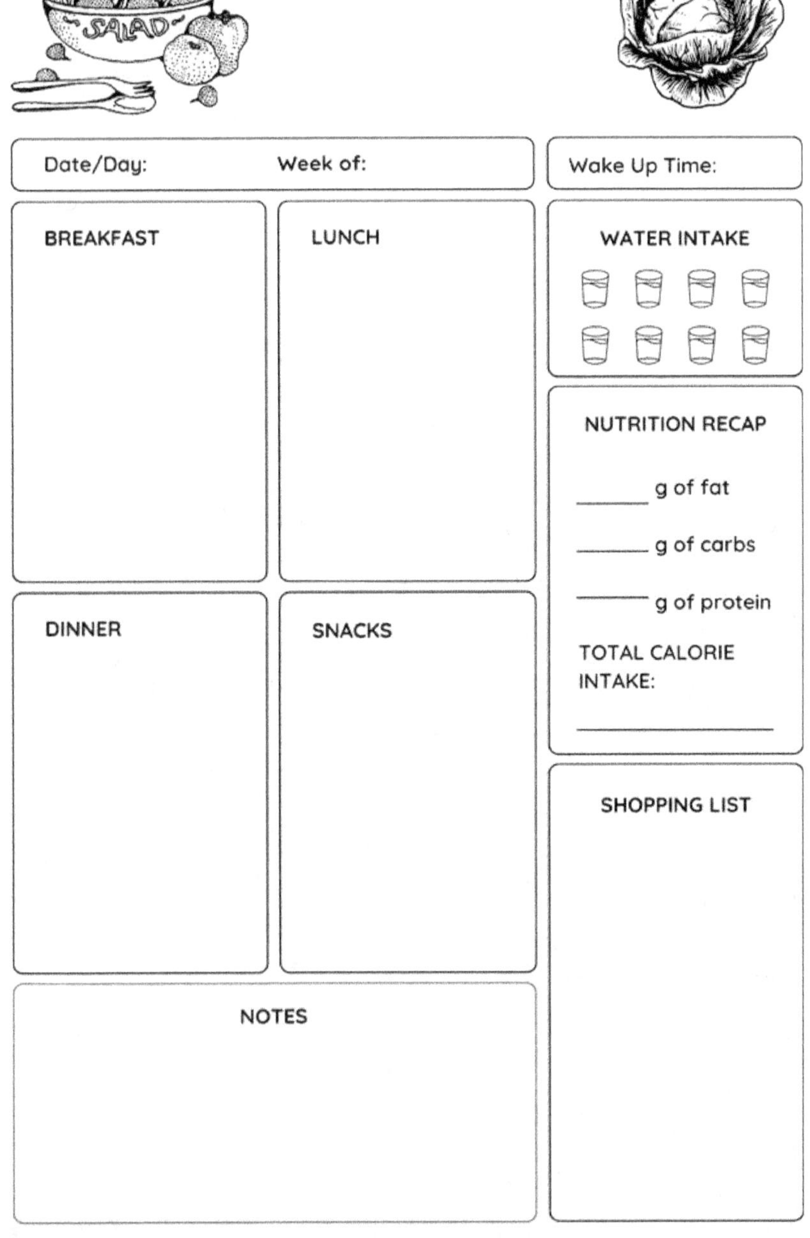

Date/Day:
Week of:
Wake Up Time:
BREAKFAST
LUNCH
WATER INTAKE
NUTRITION RECAP
_______ g of fat
_______ g of carbs
_______ g of protein
TOTAL CALORIE
INTAKE:
____
DINNER
SNACKS
SHOPPING LIST
NOTES

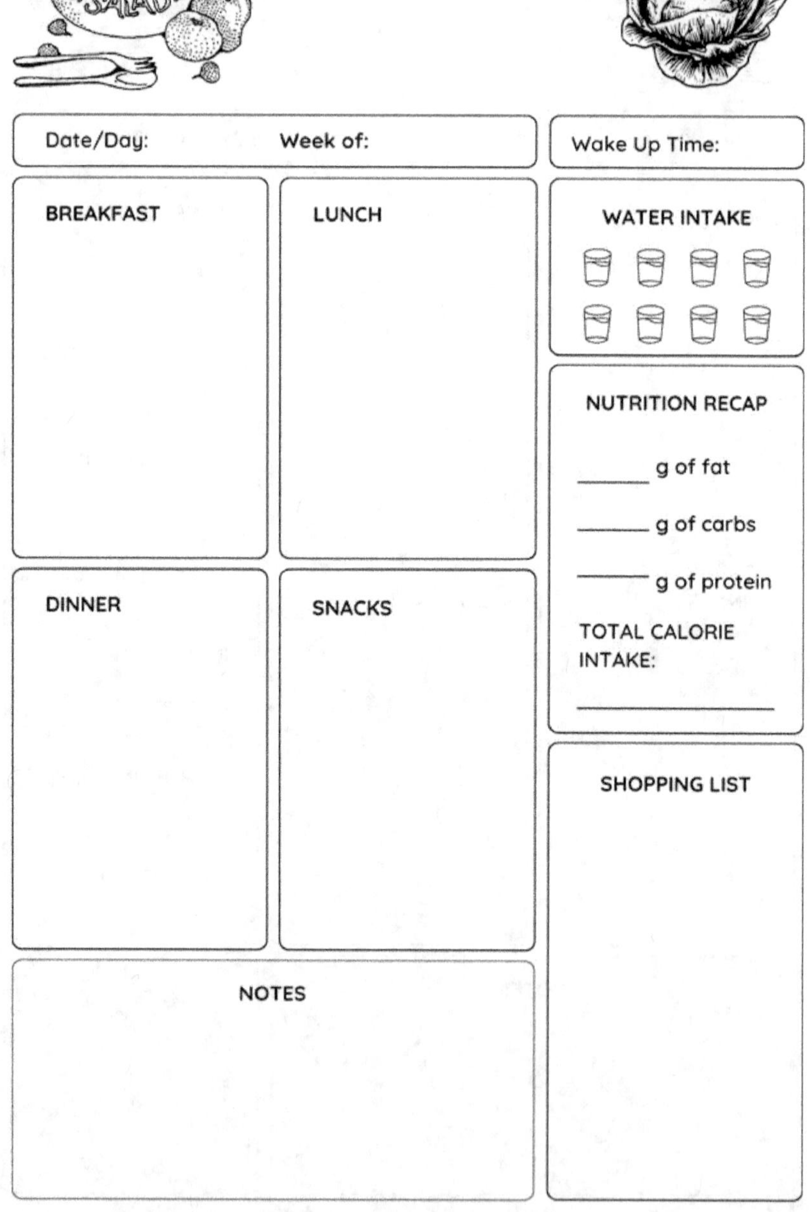

Date/Day:
Week of:
Wake Up Time:
BREAKFAST
LUNCH
WATER INTAKE
DINNER
SNACKS
NUTRITION RECAP
_______ g of fat
_______ g of carbs
_______ g of protein
TOTAL CALORIE INTAKE:
SHOPPING LIST
NOTES

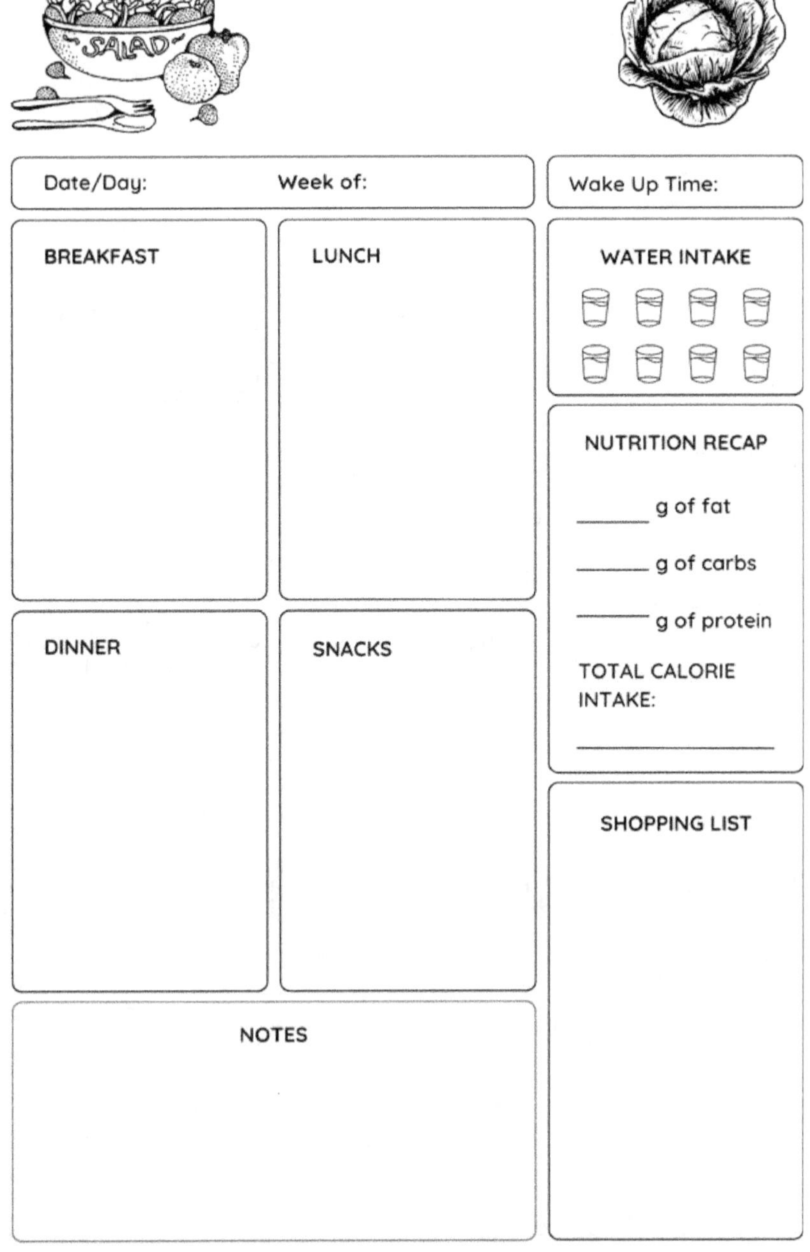

| Date/Day: | Week of: | Wake Up Time: |

BREAKFAST

LUNCH

WATER INTAKE

DINNER

SNACKS

NUTRITION RECAP

_______ g of fat

_______ g of carbs

_______ g of protein

TOTAL CALORIE INTAKE:

____

SHOPPING LIST

NOTES

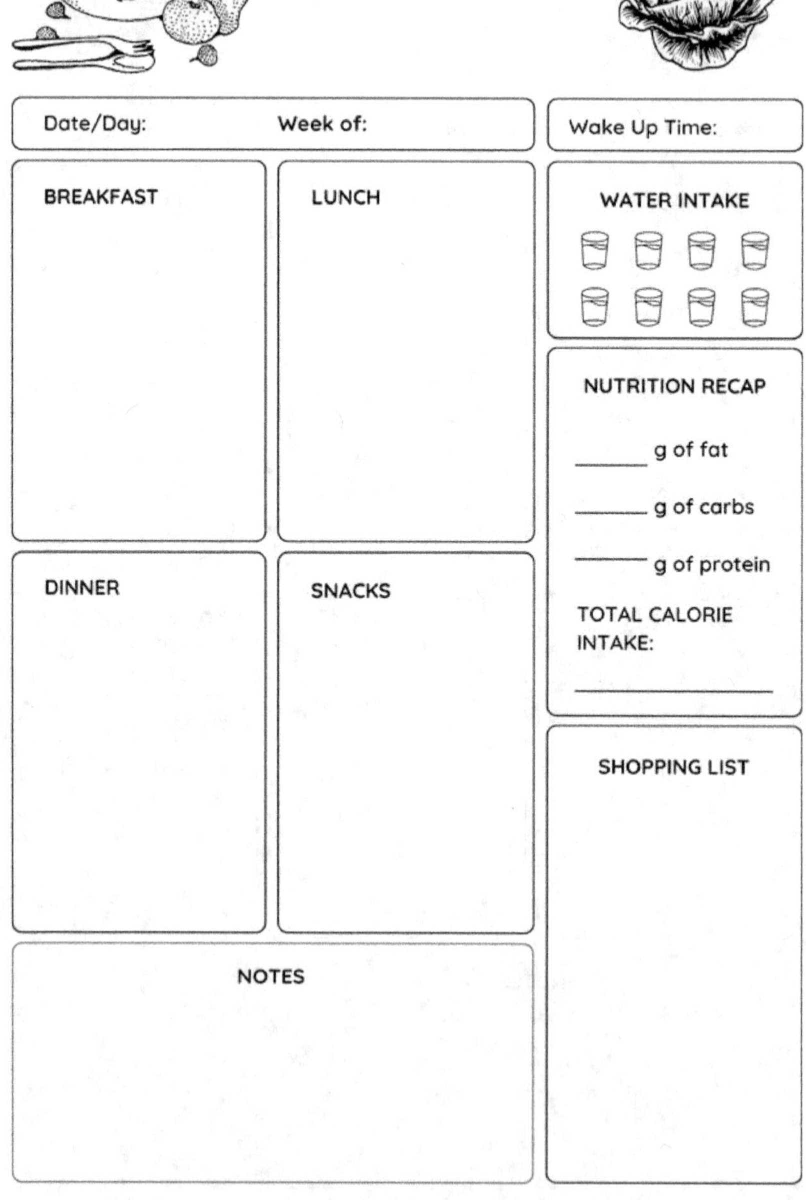

Date/Day: Week of:
Wake Up Time:
BREAKFAST
LUNCH
WATER INTAKE
NUTRITION RECAP
_______ g of fat
_______ g of carbs
_______ g of protein
TOTAL CALORIE INTAKE:
DINNER
SNACKS
SHOPPING LIST
NOTES

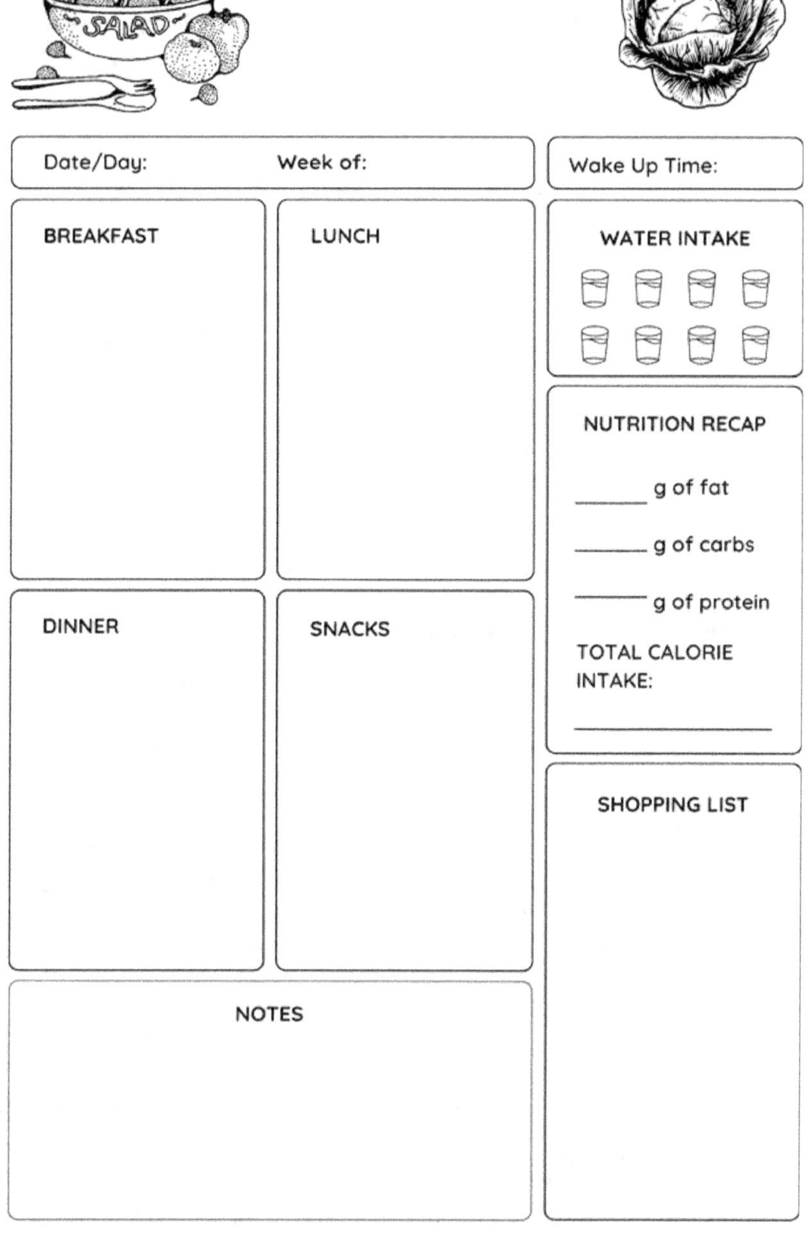

| Date/Day: | Week of: | Wake Up Time: |

BREAKFAST

LUNCH

WATER INTAKE

NUTRITION RECAP

_________ g of fat

_________ g of carbs

_________ g of protein

TOTAL CALORIE INTAKE:

____

DINNER

SNACKS

SHOPPING LIST

NOTES

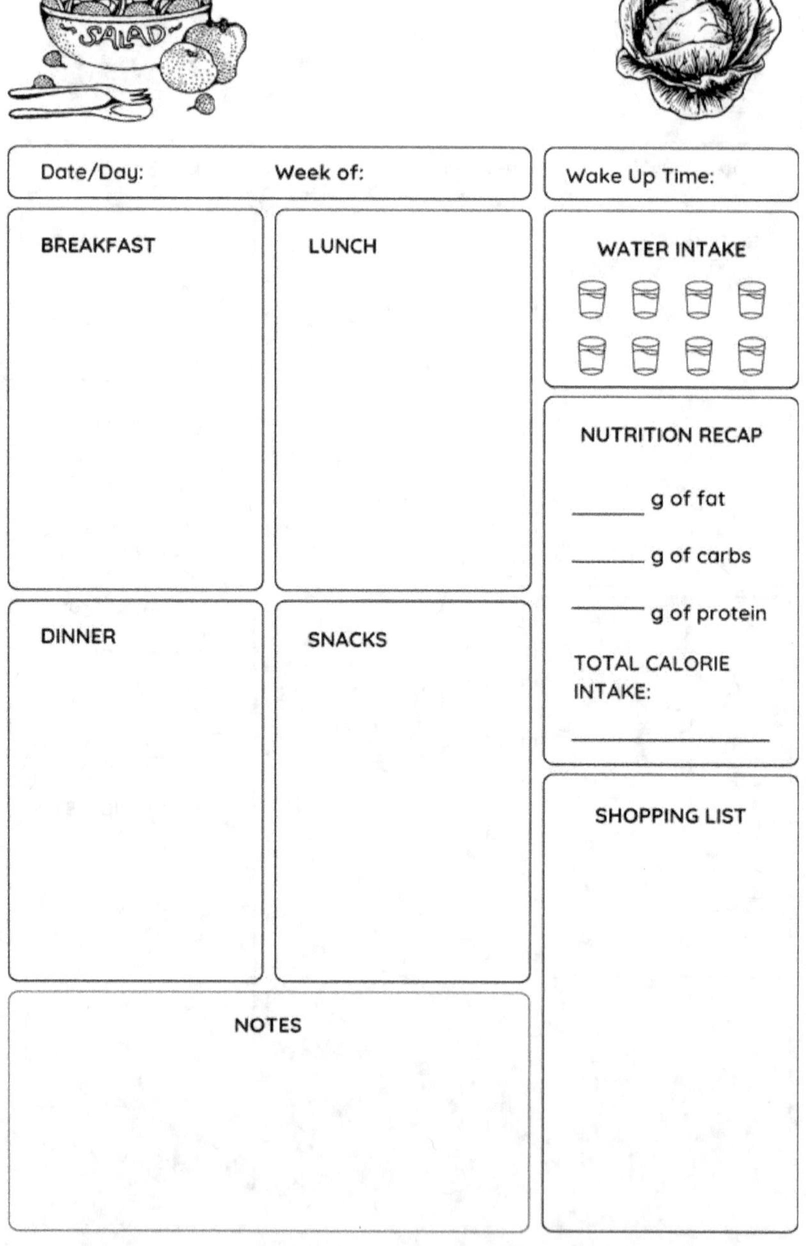

Date/Day:
Week of:
Wake Up Time:
BREAKFAST
LUNCH
WATER INTAKE
NUTRITION RECAP
_______ g of fat
_______ g of carbs
_______ g of protein
TOTAL CALORIE INTAKE:
DINNER
SNACKS
SHOPPING LIST
NOTES

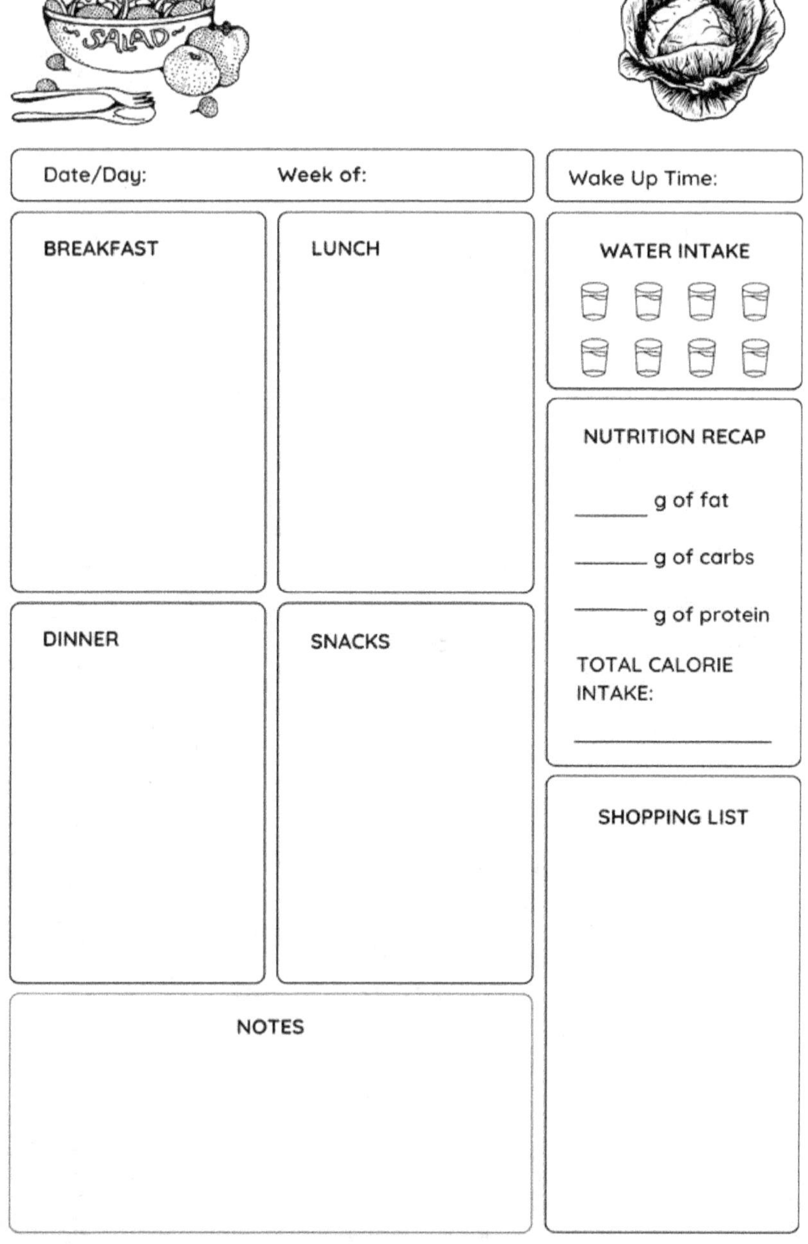

| Date/Day: | Week of: | Wake Up Time: |

BREAKFAST

LUNCH

WATER INTAKE

NUTRITION RECAP

_______ g of fat

_______ g of carbs

_______ g of protein

TOTAL CALORIE INTAKE:

____

DINNER

SNACKS

SHOPPING LIST

NOTES

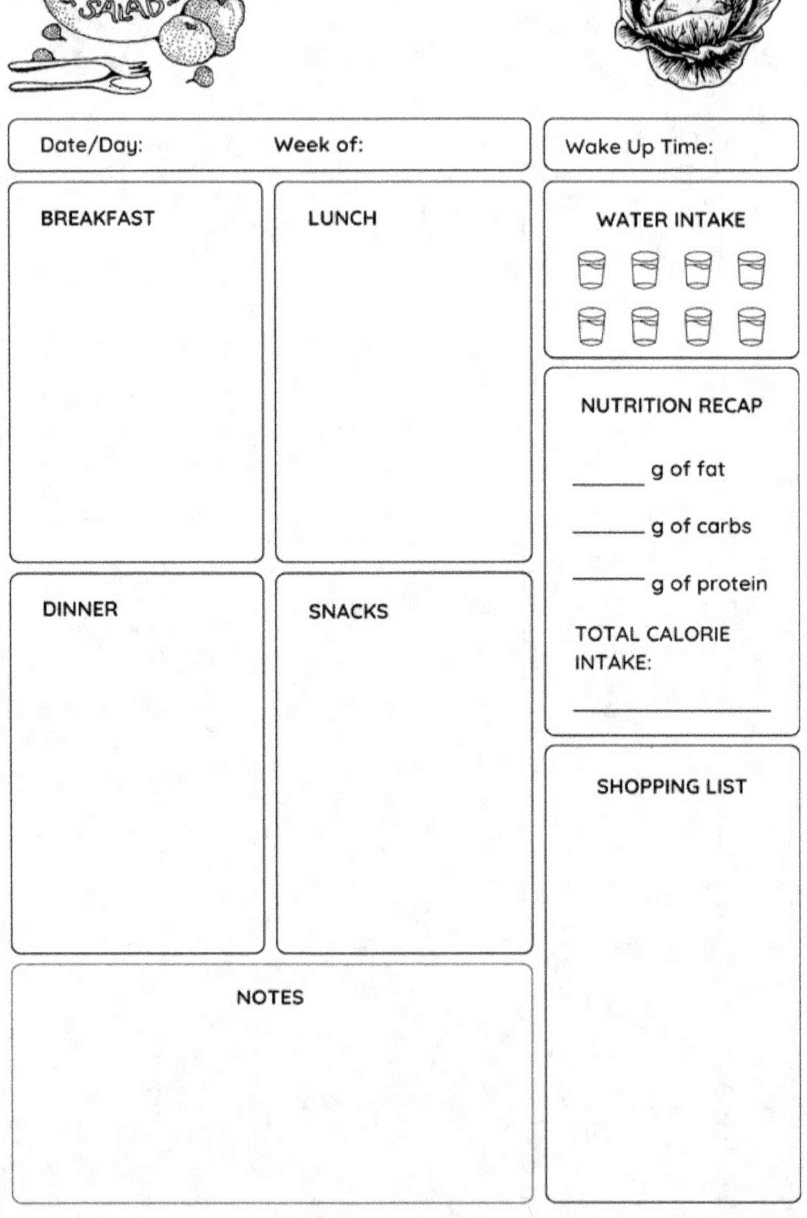

| Date/Day: | Week of: | Wake Up Time: |

BREAKFAST

LUNCH

WATER INTAKE

NUTRITION RECAP

_________ g of fat

_________ g of carbs

_________ g of protein

TOTAL CALORIE INTAKE:

____

DINNER

SNACKS

SHOPPING LIST

NOTES

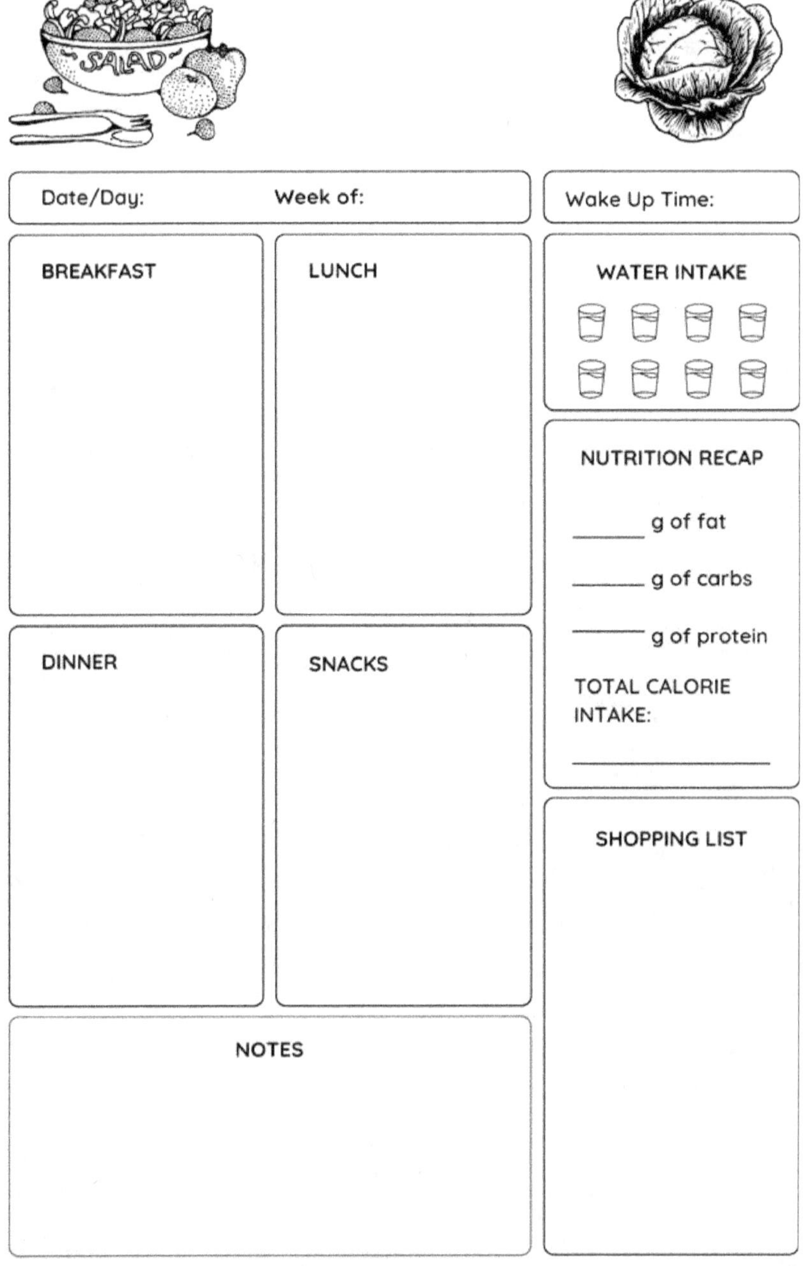

Date/Day: Week of:

Wake Up Time:

BREAKFAST

LUNCH

WATER INTAKE

NUTRITION RECAP

_______ g of fat

_______ g of carbs

_______ g of protein

TOTAL CALORIE INTAKE:

____

DINNER

SNACKS

SHOPPING LIST

NOTES

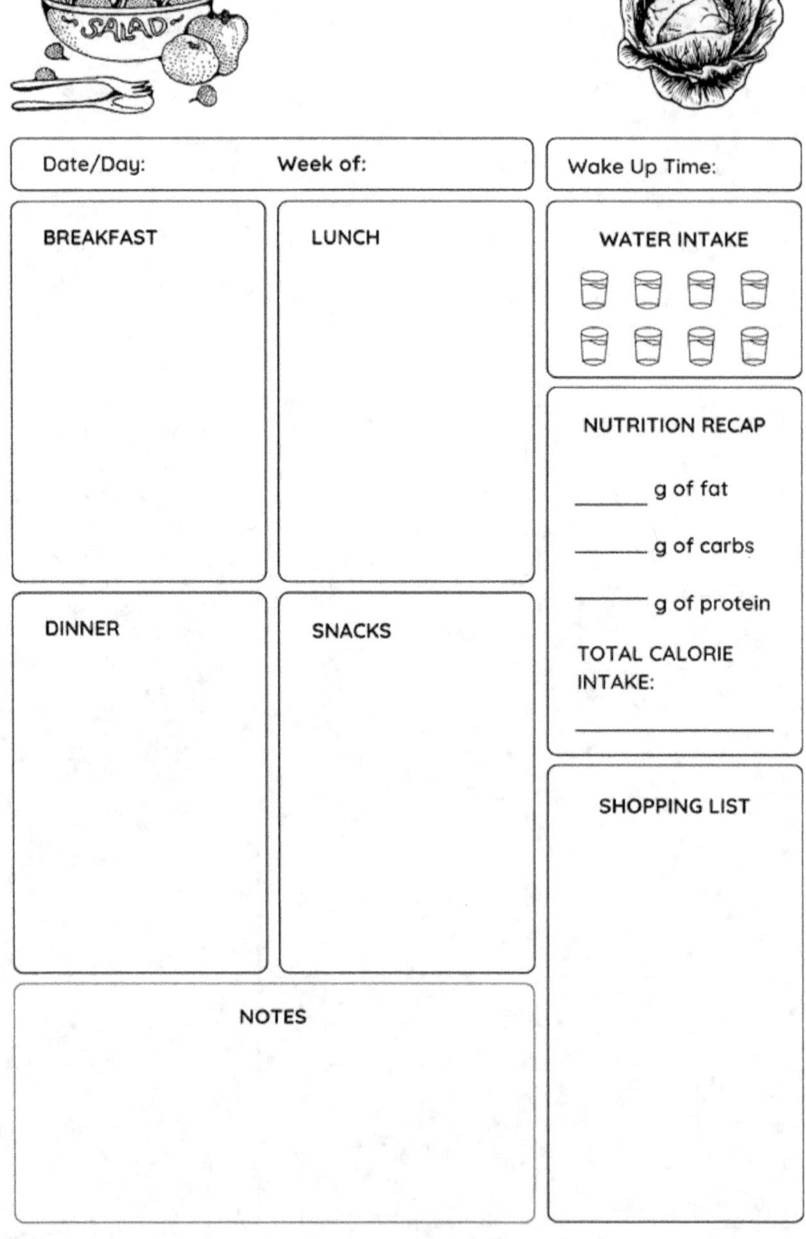

Date/Day:
Week of:
Wake Up Time:
BREAKFAST
LUNCH
WATER INTAKE
NUTRITION RECAP
_______ g of fat
_______ g of carbs
_______ g of protein
TOTAL CALORIE
INTAKE:
____
DINNER
SNACKS
SHOPPING LIST
NOTES

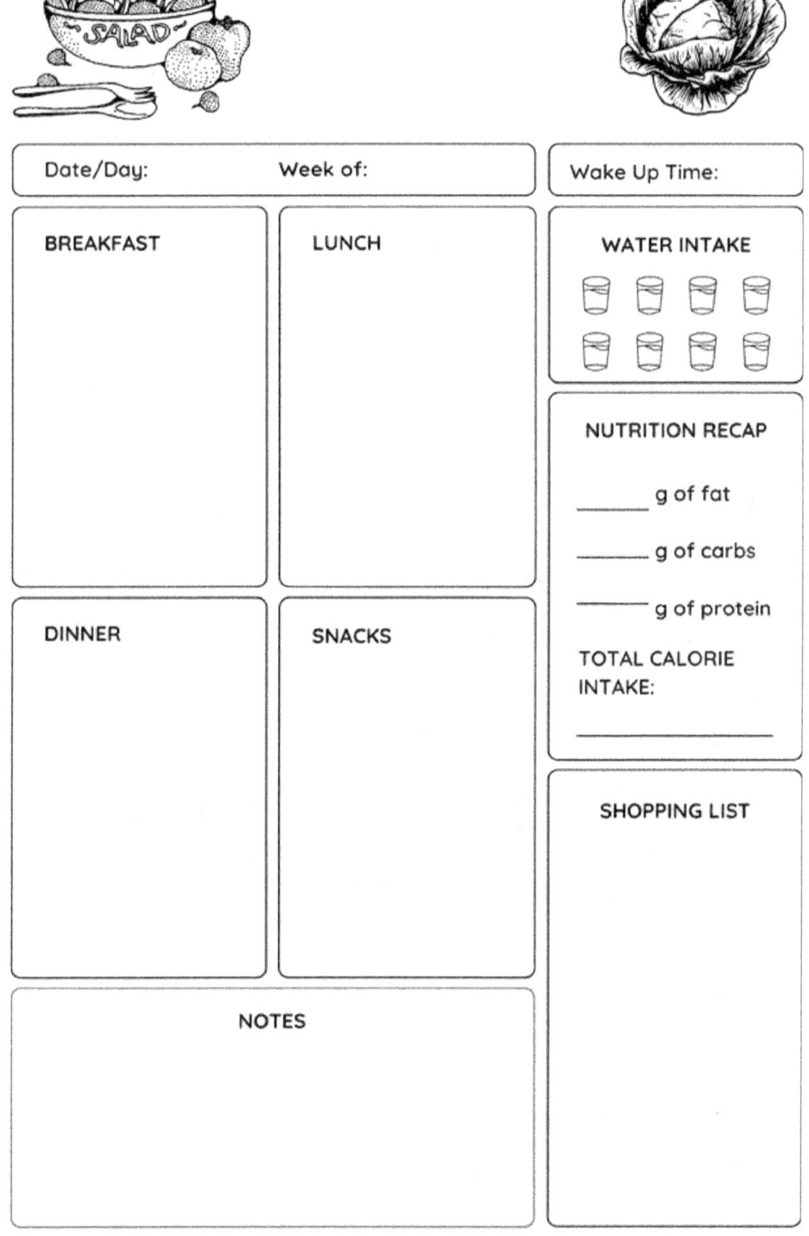

Date/Day:
Week of:
Wake Up Time:
BREAKFAST
LUNCH
WATER INTAKE
NUTRITION RECAP
________ g of fat
________ g of carbs
________ g of protein
TOTAL CALORIE INTAKE:
DINNER
SNACKS
SHOPPING LIST
NOTES

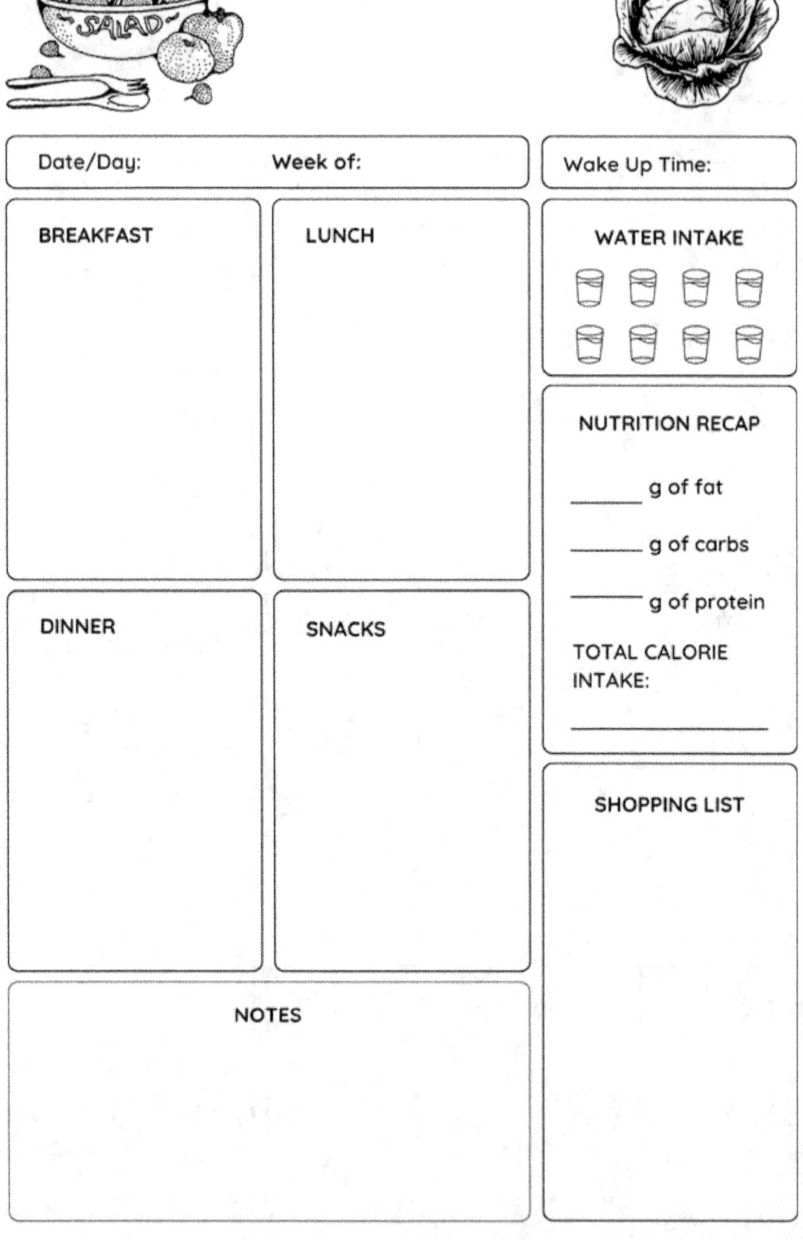
Date/Day:
Week of:
Wake Up Time:
BREAKFAST
LUNCH
WATER INTAKE
NUTRITION RECAP
_______ g of fat
_______ g of carbs
_______ g of protein
TOTAL CALORIE INTAKE:
DINNER
SNACKS
SHOPPING LIST
NOTES